No. 1 in the ┌ ┘ ┐sing Health Information series

Series Editor
Michael Rigby

WITHDRAWN
FROM STOCK

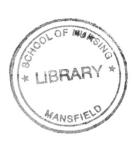

Information for Evidence-based Care

Ruth Roberts

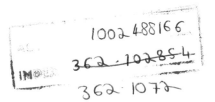
Radcliffe Medical Press

Radcliffe Medical Press
18 Marcham Road, Abingdon, Oxon OX14 1AA

British Library Cataloguing in Publication Data

A catalogue record for this book is available from the British Library.

ISBN 1 85775 356 9

Typeset by Joshua Associates Ltd, Oxford
Printed and bound by TJ International Ltd, Padstow, Cornwall

100 2488166

Contents

Series Editor's Preface

Information for Evidence-based Care

Information is a key resource in health and healthcare, but all too frequently it is seen as a challenge rather than an asset. Too often clinicians and support staff feel they are having to supply to others information of limited value, but when they themselves want information it is difficult to obtain. The whole wealth of information in the health sector can seem overwhelming yet inaccessible.

The purpose of this new series is to assist people in *Harnessing Health Information*. Information is there to be used, but that requires understanding of the information need related to the task in hand and the relevant sources. The series will build up a range of volumes addressing specific health activities and information sources.

Given its importance, in terms of policy but much more so in terms of the core mission of delivering appropriate and effective care, it is most fitting that the launch volume should be *Information for Evidence-based Care*. It addresses the very issue which should be in every clinician's and manager's mind, and therefore on the agenda of all information staff.

Ruth Roberts brings to this subject significant experience as a health professional who has implemented systematic and evidence-based practice in several parts of the United Kingdom, and led the innovative development of an applied clinical informatics system. She has undertaken personal research and teaching in information and effectiveness, and this has taken her as far afield as North America and Australia.

Evidence-based care, like so many health innovations, has started from a sound concept, been developed and promoted through specialist initiatives, and become the perceived solution to all clinical decisions. And in that process, again like so many other good ideas, it has been oversold as an instant panacea which was never intended. Thus, in a short space of time the concept has become almost threatening, the sources of advice can seem to be confusing and conflicting, yet the desired information can seem difficult to find or relate to daily practice. Moreover, the evidence cannot give a treatment plan for an individual patient – it is there to aid and inform the clinician, not to give directions.

In *Information for Evidence-based Care* Ruth Roberts sets the context by mapping concisely the origins of the concept, and how it has become embedded into NHS policy and on into common parlance. Definition of what can be considered as 'evidence', and its recognised quality levels, leads on to consideration of the sources of information available to clinicians, and how to access them. It is important to recognise that available information is only as good as its robustness, and its relevance to the specific issue, and therefore critical appraisal and resolution of conflict are addressed fully. Approaches to guideline development, and the role of patient involvement, lead into the key issue – how to get evidence into practice. The concluding theme is that there is no end point – self-review and audit, and a culture of continual monitoring of external and internal information-based evidence, are the essentials of constantly updated evidence-based care in practice.

This new series will only be successful if it enables health information to be more easily harnessed in practice. Evidence will only get into the support of care if the information sources are understood and accessed. I hope that *Information for Evidence-based Care* really does improve healthcare by improving practice in *Harnessing Health Information*.

Michael Rigby
May 1999

About the author

Ruth Roberts RCN, SCM, MSC is Lecturer at the School of Post-graduate Studies in Medical and Health Care, Swansea. She undertook her general nurse training at the Queen Elizabeth Hospital, Birmingham (where she was awarded the Gold Medal for general training), and then qualified in midwifery in Bristol and Exeter. After that she specialised in care of the elderly, and from her initial appointment as ward sister sought to ensure that practice was evidence based.

Progressing through a series of senior nursing positions in South East England largely related to service innovation, including secondment as Regional Nursing Process Co-ordinator to South West Thames Region to facilitate the strengthening of the systematic approach to nursing throughout that region, she was then appointed to Cambridge Health Authority as Nurse Consultant – Services for the Elderly, the first nurse consultant post in the UK. During this time she was a member of the Open University team which in 1984 produced the first distance learning material in the UK for qualified nurses, *A Systematic Approach to Nursing Care: An Introduction*.

Her commitment to innovation in information-based practice then took her to Wales, as project leader to develop a prototype Clinical Nursing Information System, an essential aspect of which was the encapsulated clinical knowledge base. She then became Nursing Information Systems Project Manager for Wales, reporting professionally to the Chief Nursing Officer for Wales.

In her current position she undertakes a range of teaching and research activities. This includes organising the School's innovative MSc course in Clinical Audit and Effectiveness, and involvement in a number of national projects in Wales and England, and in European projects. Simultaneously, she has continued her own studies, gaining her MSc in Health Information Management at the University of Wales, Aberystwyth, and is now studying clinical education methodology at Cardiff. She has published widely on clinical information systems, the nursing process and care of the elderly, and has presented a number of papers at national and international expert conferences.

1 History of evidence-based care

All clinicians want to practice well, and seek to base their decisions and care on the best possible knowledge. However, it is not always easy to keep up-to-date as new information about the value of current practices and alternatives becomes available almost daily. It is difficult for healthcare practitioners to manage this deluge of information, let alone review the information and decide what changes in practice are required. It has been estimated that there are over 20 000 medical journals, and over two million articles published each year;[1] and that a doctor practising general medicine would need to read 19 articles every single day in a year just to keep abreast with the publications.[2]

There are inevitably delays between the publication of any scientific research and its adoption, and there are concerns about the significant delay in clinicians using information from research in the clinical setting. Delayed uptake of the results of research findings is not new; in 1601 James Lancaster showed the effectiveness of using lemon juice to prevent scurvy. Nearly 150 years later, James Lind undertook a similar experiment, and the British navy eventually adopted the prophylactic at the start of the 19th century. More recently, thrombolytic treatment for myocardial infarction was shown to be clinically effective more than a decade before it became widely advocated.

Nowadays there are many patients who have access to the Internet and other electronic databases, and these patients are starting to use that information to query health professionals' decisions about their healthcare. Many health professionals welcome this changing culture, whilst at the same time expressing their concerns about their own limited access to relevant up-to-date journals, review publications and databases. Many health professionals also express concern about their limited awareness of where to look, their lack of skills in quickly finding, retrieving and appraising relevant published information so that they can review the care they give to patients, and balancing the time required to undertake this and still provide care. For those who are feeling overwhelmed about where to start and what to do, this book aims to provide some information about evidence-based care and pointers to further sources.

Professional developments

During the mid-1980s McMaster Medical School, Canada, commenced problem-based, self-directed education for both under-graduate and postgraduate medical students; this approach was intended to promote life-long learning and the phrase 'evidence-based medicine' (EBM) was originally established at McMaster. Evidence-based medicine has been defined as 'the conscientious, explicit, and judicious use of current best evidence in making decisions about the care of individual patients'.[3] There have been concerns that this approach places too much emphasis on the science of medicine and tends to ignore the art of medicine. In response, the evidence-based medicine community has argued that practising evidence-based medicine involves integrating individual clinical experience with the best available external evidence and patients' choice, and that it is an enhancement, rather than a replacement, of traditional skills. When practising evidence-based medicine doctors turn clinical problems into questions and then systematically locate, appraise and use research findings as the basis for clinical decisions. The United Kingdom has been able to benefit from the pioneering McMaster approach through the appointment of David Sackett as Director of the UK's first Centre for Evidence-based Medicine, which is based in Oxford.

In the UK, Cochrane had raised questions as to the degree to which medical practice was based on robust research. A large proportion of practice had not been particularly well evaluated and many of the most commonly used therapies and procedures were not necessarily those shown, by research, to be the most suitable. In his publication *Efficiency and Effectiveness*,[4] he argued that more needed to be known about the benefits and costs of clinical activities in order to achieve optimum results from the NHS.

Nurses and the professions allied to medicine have been practising using a problem oriented approach since the early 1980s. When considering the possible actions to take in relation to each identified problem, nurses were encouraged to take into account priorities, constraints and resources, but it was also emphasised that 'nursing practice should be based on sound research evidence'.[5] However a study, reported on in 1993,[6] found that there were still difficulties with incorporating research findings into nursing practice, with only 21% of the group investigated having implemented a new research finding during the previous six months. Another study identified that nurses seeking information on patient care tended to require quick decision making and sought directions from knowledgeable oral sources or quick reference material, rather than publications.[7]

The majority of clinical care is provided by healthcare teams, and the advocates of evidence-based medicine have stated that 'the principles, strategies and tactics of EBM are universally applicable throughout the health professions'.[8] This view appears to have been accepted by the other health professions, as can be seen by a proliferation of evidence-based professional journals and the establishment of a Centre for Evidence-based Nursing. The professional organisations are also promoting evidence-based practice; for example, the Chartered Society of Physiotherapy has played an active role in helping to enhance members' understanding of evidence-based practice, and in creating opportunities for further development of the profession's knowledge base. This interest by all healthcare professionals has also been accompanied by the adoption of the phrase 'evidence-based healthcare' which has been described by Appleby et al. as:

> a shift in the culture of healthcare provision away from basing decisions on opinion, past practice and precedent towards making more use of science, research and evidence to guide decision making. It requires the evaluation of the effectiveness of medical interventions, the dissemination of the results of evaluation and finally the application of those findings to practice.[9]

Practising evidence-based healthcare does not just involve browsing journals to keep up-to-date. Clinicians need to have access to library facilities and good information seeking and retrieval skills, as well as the motivation to systematically obtain information. Clinicians will also need to have sufficient knowledge of research design and methods to decide which studies to take into account and which to dismiss. A clinician's capacity to make evidence-based decisions will also be limited to the extent that the organisation facilitates and supports such decisions.

Policy impact and development

Since its inception, in 1948, the core purpose of the National Health Service (NHS) has been to secure improvement in the physical and mental health of the population. The NHS was intended to deliver healthcare in a rational, efficient and fair way across the UK and to be free at the point of delivery. In 1983, the Griffiths Inquiry identified that 'clinical evaluation of particular practices is by no means common, and the economic evaluation of those practices [is] extremely rare'.[10] This concern at policy level built on the professional concerns of Cochrane and others as already described.

Quality of healthcare

Quality of healthcare became an explicit issue in the health reforms immediately after the Griffiths Inquiry. The Confidential Enquiry into Perioperative Deaths[11] highlighted, graphically, the adverse effects of not using best practice and was a major stimulant to audit, and the 1989 reforms introduced obligatory medical audit in acute care. The emphasis on quality and audit could be considered as being the beginning of the NHS's interests in evidence-based practice. Under Section 62 of the *National Health Service and Community Care Act 1990*, an independent source of expert advice on standards on clinical care, and access to and availability of services, for NHS patients was established. The Clinical Standards Advisory Group (CSAG) provides advice to UK Health Ministers and the NHS; its members are nominated by the medical, nursing and dental Royal Colleges and their faculties, and the organisations of the professions allied to medicine. The Chairs of the Standing Medical, Nursing and Midwifery, and Dental Advisory Committees are also members. The Clinical Standards Advisory Group remits are set by the Health Ministers in discussion with the group.

Managing resources

Concentrating resources on key priorities, identifying the most effective interventions and ensuring that they were translated into practice became the major themes in most health policy documents during the 1980s and 1990s. The UK has not been alone in taking these themes, as worldwide the needs and demands for healthcare are increasing at a faster rate than the increase in resources available to provide it. Improved information has been an important element of the UK strategies, with the information intended to be of use to clinicians and health service managers in monitoring progress.

Research and development

The role of research and development became more focused during the early 1990s following a House of Lords Select Committee on Science and Technology report which stated that 'the NHS should articulate its needs [for research]; it should assist in meeting those needs; and it should ensure that the fruits of research are systematically transferred into service'.[12] England was the first of the four UK countries to appoint an NHS Director of Research and Development (R&D), and England published its first R&D strategy in 1991. The four countries' initial research strategies were aimed at creating an evaluation culture within the NHS and promoting the use and exchange of existing research. Following the publication of England's strategy, information dissemination systems were established; these included the UK Cochrane Centre (1992), the NHS Centre for Reviews and Dissemination (1994) and the NHS R&D Projects Register System. The Cochrane Centre, the Cochrane Library and the NHS Centre for Reviews and Dissemination are discussed in Chapter 4.

The NHS Projects Register System is a computer-based project register of funded research projects. The register is intended to support efficient research management by identifying unwanted research duplication in NHS research and to provide information for NHS managers commissioning new research or using existing research. The projects register also provides input to research reviews and meta-analyses. Each of the four UK countries maintains a register.

Making more use of science, research and evidence to guide decision making in healthcare has evolved through the healthcare professions and through the development of health policy. Evidence-based healthcare involves turning clinical problems into questions and then systematically locating, appraising and using the best available research evidence as the basis for clinical practice. Sometimes the terms 'evidence-based care' and 'clinical effectiveness' are used to mean the same – however, these terms are not synonymous and Chapter 2 focuses on clinical effectiveness and highlights why the terms should not be used to mean the same.

References

1   Haines A (1996) The science of perpetual change. *British Journal of General Practice.* **46**: 115–19.

2   Davidoff F, Haynes B, Sackett D *et al.* (1995) Evidence-based medicine. *British Medical Journal.* **310**: 1085–6.

3   Sackett DL, Rosenberg WMC, Muir Gray JA, Haynes RB and Richardson WS (1996) Evidence based medicine: what it is and what it isn't. *British Medical Journal.* **312**: 71–2.

4   Cochrane AL (1972) *Efficiency and effectiveness: random reflections on health services.* London: Nuffield Provincial Hospitals Trust and British Medical Journal, London. Reprinted in revised format, 1989.

5   Binnie A, Bond S, Law G *et al.* (1984) *A Systematic Approach to Nursing Care: an introduction.* The Open University Press, Milton Keynes.

6   Bostrom J and Sutter WN (1993) Research utilisation: making the link to practice. *Journal of Nursing Staff Development.* **9**: 28–34.

7   Blythe J and Royle J (1993) Assessing nurses' information needs in the work environment. *Bulletin of Medical Libraries Association.* **81**(4): 433–5.

8   Sackett DL, Richardson WS, Rosenberg W and Haynes RB (1997) *Evidence-based Medicine: how to practice & teach EBM.* Churchill Livingstone, Edinburgh.

9   Appleby J, Walshe K and Ham C (1995) *Acting on the Evidence: a review of clinical effectiveness sources of information, dissemination and implementation.* NAHAT Research Paper 17. NAHAT, Birmingham.

10 Department of Health and Social Security (1983) *NHS Management Inquiry: Griffiths NHS Management Inquiry report.* Department of Health and Social Security, London.

11 Buck N, Devlin HB and Lunn JN (1987) *The Report of a Confidential Enquiry into Perioperative Death.* The Nuffield Provincial Hospitals Trust, London.

12 House of Lords Select Committee on Science and Technology (1988) *Priorities in Medical Research: 3rd Report, Session 1987–88.* HMSO, London.

2 Clinical effectiveness and NHS policy

Clinical effectiveness became a major agenda item in the late 1990s. The concept behind the clinical effectiveness initiative was that:

> the NHS as an institution, and clinicians as autonomous professionals, should abandon apparently ineffective treatments and should promote instead those of proven value to patients. By doing so, the outcome of the provision of health care on the nation's health would be improved, even within existing resources.[1]

Clinical effectiveness involves considerations of financial efficiency – however, the practice of evidence-based care 'to maximise the quality and quantity of life for individual patients . . . may raise rather than lower the cost of their care'.[2]

Clinical effectiveness strategies have been adopted by the four countries of the United Kingdom. These have similar aims, but there have been differences in the way each country has approached the task.

England

In England the initiative has been a more central approach, with the Department of Health incorporating the development and delivery of clinically effective services into priority setting and planning guidelines. Executive letters were used to inform health authorities and trusts about the principles of the initiative and sources of information. The initial definition of clinical effectiveness came from the NHS Executive and included consideration of financial efficiency; the extent that an intervention can 'secure the greatest possible health gain from the available resources'[3] has been re-iterated in later Executive letters.

The first Executive letter commended seven clinical guidelines that had been evaluated on behalf of the NHS Management Executive. For the year 1995/96 health authorities were requested to move investment into two specific areas for which good evidence of effectiveness was available, and away from two areas of care that had been shown to be less effective. Health authorities could decide for themselves what these areas should be.

Promoting Clinical Effectiveness[4] outlined a framework for action under three headings: inform, change and monitor. It was targeted at chief executives of health authorities and NHS trusts, plus clinicians responsible for developing strategies for clinical effectiveness. The section on change highlighted initiatives such as clinical audit, guidelines, education and training, and the provision of better information to patients, as methods of ensuring that clinical effectiveness information became incorporated into practice. The use of existing data sets, for example Health Service Indicators, Public Health Common Data Sets and Population Health Outcome Indicators, were highlighted in the section on monitoring the changes in clinical practice and the resultant health and clinical outcomes. It was also proposed that other data sets currently being developed, such as *Health of the Nation* measures, NHS Performance Measures, Clinical Indicators and Indicators based on Primary Care and Prescription Data, would be used for monitoring. Other long-term development programmes, such as the Clinical Terms Project, Health Benefit Groups, *Health of the Nation* Outcomes Scales and the Information Management and Technology Strategy, were intended to improve the routine collection of complete, good quality data to monitor clinical effectiveness. National audits would provide national analyses of variations in practice and could be a starting point for local review of effective care. Clinical effectiveness performance development frameworks were to be implemented by Regional Offices of the Executive to support the programme in England.

Promoting the use of research within the NHS was one of the key aims of the NHS R&D strategy. Oxford Regional Health Authority established a project – Getting Research into Purchasing and Practice (GRiPP) – which took a proactive approach to promoting vigorously the new knowledge derived from research. Five therapeutic interventions were selected – these were ones for which there was good research of effectiveness and it was known that there was a gap between what was known and what was practised. The project found that by focusing on these specific treatments, the concepts of evidence-based decision making and the need to use evidence in all decisions were adopted much more quickly than 'if general exhortations to practice evidence-based decision making had been made'.[5]

Wales

Towards Evidence Based Practice: a clinical effectiveness initiative for Wales[6] provides the three year strategic framework for Wales and was developed following five preliminary workshops across Wales and in meetings of the Clinical Effectiveness Group. This group was established in 1994, under the chairmanship of the Chief Medical Officer for Wales, with the Chief Nursing Officer for Wales as vice-chair and three quarters of the membership from the clinical professions. Other members are from management, academic departments and Community Health Councils. The clinical effect-iveness initiative was launched by the Secretary of State for Wales in May 1995 with the objective that 'all health care staff work together and in partnership with patients to increase the proportion of clinical services shown by evidence to be effective'.[6] The initiative was based on four principles:

- practice should be based on sound evidence of effectiveness
- the patient's view of the outcome of treatment or care should be given significant weight
- R&D, education, audit, and information programmes should support the new emphasis on evidence and on the patient perspective
- more attention should be given to setting standards and assessing achievement.

The focus of the initiative was on helping those who provide care to acquire the skills, information and resources they needed to be clinically effective. Clinical teams were encouraged to look critically at their own situation in terms of available skills, audit practice and access to information, and a checklist to undertake this was included in the document.[6] The Clinical Effectiveness Group held expert workshops to discuss the three main themes of the initiative:

- improving access to evidence and information
- helping practitioners acquire the knowledge and skills to use that evidence
- and ensuring that working arrangements support effective care.

Briefing documents were produced on each of these themes.[7–9] Local areas were also asked to review how people in different parts of the service could work together to develop new approaches, for example by developing existing audit and continuing education structures.

Already in 1989 the *Strategic Intent and Direction for the NHS in Wales*[10] had identified that health gain was the key criterion for judging the effectiveness of NHS Wales. Prior to the publication of this document work had been undertaken on producing multi-disciplinary protocols for investment in health gain. These summarised current views on effectiveness in 12 important areas, including mental distress and illness, mental handicap, cancers, cardiovascular diseases, respiratory diseases, physical disability and discomfort, and maternity and early child health. Work on these continued as part of the clinical effectiveness initiative and the development of guidelines was also proposed.

The Clinical Effectiveness Support Unit (CESU) was established in 1995 to provide practical support to health professionals throughout Wales, the Clinical Effectiveness Group and its subgroups. The subgroups were set up to monitor and accelerate progress on key aspects of the initiative, such as clinical audit, use of outcome measures and the investigation of new methods of information dissemination.

The three year initiative on clinical effectiveness has now ended, and a review of progress has been undertaken. CESU supported five national demonstration projects which have all produced changes in local practice. Reports from these projects have been widely circulated throughout the Principality. In addition, over 100 local projects have been centrally funded which have tried to improve local working or generate new information to guide practice. The Clinical Effectiveness Newsletter reports on progress throughout the Principality and encourages the sharing of ideas and examples in order to engender participation. Over 2000 people have received some training on clinical effectiveness and several hundred have received an introduction to critical appraisal skills. Five large-scale national audits have been undertaken, and the colorectal cancer audit has already changed aspects of practice. Although the initiative has reached the end of its three year programme, work is continuing to help practitioners acquire the skills, information and resources they need to be clinically effective.

Scotland

Scotland established a five year development programme, the focus being on the production of guidelines. Twelve guidelines were identified for inclusion in the 1995/96 contracts – these included the management of acute myocardial infarction; management of stroke; drug treatment of peripheral vascular disease; indications for tonsil-lectomy; and interface between hospital and community develop-ment of a generic discharge summary. A common core programme was aimed at reducing duplication of effort, co-ordinating local and national work and restricting imperatives to a manageable number. Clear criteria were used to determine the activities, and the limitation ensured that not only was there adequate funding, but also that they would be implemented in routine clinical practice.

An integrated and clearly defined structure was established in which the roles and relationships among the many organisations involved with clinical effectiveness have been defined. The Clinical Resources Audit Group (CRAG) provided a forum for assessing the effective and efficient use of clinical resources and stimulated the development of guidelines, outcome indicators and clinical audit.[11] It disseminated information on these topics and supports the Scottish Audit Resource Centre. National clinical guidelines are produced by the Scottish Intercollegiate Guidelines Network (SIGN), a grouping of Royal Colleges and other medical and professional bodies. The Scottish Health Purchasing Information Centre (SHPIC) assesses relevant information on the clinical and cost-effectiveness of specific healthcare interventions, and the Scottish Needs Assessment Pro-gramme (SNAP) co-ordinates the work of the public health departments in assessing the healthcare needs of the population. The commissioning of research on a range of conditions, metho-dologies, new developments and techniques is undertaken by the Chief Scientist's Office, which also supports a number of research units and maintains a database of completed research work.

Northern Ireland

Promotion of effectiveness in health and social care, dissemination of information and promotion of the implementation of good practice in agreed priority areas is the remit of the Departmental Clinical Effectiveness Group of the Department of Health and Personal Social Services. The group is co-chaired by the Chief Medical and

Nursing Officers for Northern Ireland and was established in 1997. The Clinical Resource Efficiency Support Group produces and publishes reports and guidelines on two or three key practice or service areas each year and a regional database holds data on audit and related projects. The Northern Ireland Research and Development Office was established in 1997 to commission new research and disseminate research findings with the aim of providing an evidence base for effective health and social care.

The recent White Papers on the new NHS and quality within the NHS have emphasised that all patients are entitled to high-quality care wherever they live and that 'clinical decisions should be based on the best possible evidence of effectiveness'.[12] There is also an emphasis that all staff should be up-to-date within their field and that there is the need for life long learning. For the first time the NHS will have a requirement to meet more than a financial statutory duty, as the NHS is now required to adopt a 'structured and coherent approach to clinical quality, placing duties and expectations on local healthcare organisations as well as individuals'.[12] The potential impact on evidence-based care is addressed in Chapter 9.

This continuing emphasis on evidence-based practice puts up-to-date information at the centre of healthcare. It means that individuals, clinical teams and organisations will need to have access to library facilities; good information seeking and retrieval skills in order to systematically obtain the evidence; skills to determine whether the evidence presented in the research papers is valid, useful and appropriate for the local situation; skills to successfully implement the proposed changes into practice; and the ability to monitor that these changes are achieving the desired outcome.

References

1   Clinical Standards Advisory Group (1998) *Clinical Effectiveness: report on clinical effectiveness using stroke care as an example.* The Stationery Office, London.
2   Sackett DL, Rosenberg WMC, Gray JAM *et al.* (1996) Evidence-based medicine: what it is and what it isn't. *British Medical Journal.* **312**: 71–2.
3   NHS Executive (1996) *Clinical Guidelines: using clinical guidelines to improve patient care within the NHS.* Department of Health, Leeds.

4   NHS Executive (1996) *Promoting Clinical Effectiveness: a framework for action in and through the NHS*. Department of Health, Leeds.

5   Muir Gray JA (1997) *Evidence-based Healthcare: how to make health policy and management decisions*. Churchill Livingstone, Edinburgh.

6   Welsh Office (1995) *Towards Evidence Based Practice*. Central Office of Information, Cardiff

7   Welsh Office (1995) *Improving Access to Evidence and Information: a clinical effectiveness initiative for Wales. Briefing Paper 1*. Welsh Office, Cardiff.

8   Welsh Office (1996) *Helping Practitioners Use the Evidence: a clinical effectiveness initiative for Wales. Briefing Paper 2*. Welsh Office, Cardiff.

9   Welsh Office (1996) *Developing the Working Environment: a clinical effectiveness initiative for Wales. Briefing Paper 3*. Welsh Office, Cardiff.

10 Welsh Office and NHS Directorate: Welsh Health Planning Forum (1989) *Strategic Intent and Direction for the NHS in Wales*. Welsh Office, Cardiff.

11 Clinical Resource and Audit Group (1993) *Clinical Guidelines: report of a working group*. Scottish Office Home and Health Department, Edinburgh.

12 Department of Health (1998) *A First Class Service: quality in the new NHS*. The Stationery Office, London.

3 Obtaining the evidence for clinical decisions

Throughout our daily lives we make numerous decisions. Any decision-making process involves collecting and analysing information in order to choose from alternatives the best way to achieve a goal or goals. Doctors mainly make clinical decisions in relation to diagnosis, estimating prognosis, assessing relevant outcomes, assessing the benefits and risks of alternative treatments, and determining the consequences of different treatment options. The main focus of clinical decision making for nurses and the professions allied to medicine is the management of patient problems and their treatment. The information to assist with clinical decision making comes from the patient, the patient's family and carers, the patient's healthcare record, results from investigations, personal knowledge, the knowledge of other members of the healthcare team, and publications. In 1996, the editor of the *British Medical Journal* claimed that 'experienced doctors use about six million pieces of information to manage their patients' and that 'about a third of doctors' time is spent recording and synthesizing information'.[1]

Clinical decision making

All health professionals have a knowledge base of healthcare. A dictionary definition of knowledge is 'the facts or experiences known by a person or group of people; the state of knowing; specific information about a subject'.[2] The initial theoretical and practical understanding of the subject of healthcare commences with the education and training of the health professional, and continuing professional development helps to keep this understanding up-to-date. Reading journals and textbooks is another way of keeping up-to-date – however, healthcare textbooks are often out of date even when new, as important new papers are published which may have an impact on the material content of the book. Over the last 20 years there have been significant scientific advances in healthcare, and there is now a deluge of healthcare information being published which makes it extremely difficult for a healthcare professional to stay up-to-date, even in their own field. There is also a limit as to how much of this information the human memory can recall at any one time.

To make clinical decisions that are based on good quality information means that health professionals need more than their own knowledge and experience of what is known, they need to access specific information about a subject and the wider facts and experiences of others. Various studies of the impact of textual information on clinical decision making by doctors have shown that information received from a library relating to current medical cases had probably changed some aspect of patient care, with one study showing that 89% of clinicians involved agreed that information provided by library and information services contributed to their clinical decision making.[3] Another study showed that physicians rated the textual information more highly than that provided by diagnostic imaging, laboratory tests and discussion with colleagues.[4]

In 1991, it was stated that 'only about 15% of medical interventions are supported by solid scientific evidence',[5] although more recent studies indicate that there are higher levels of use of scientifically validated treatments.[6,7] To practise evidence-based healthcare, health professionals need to make more use of research and evidence to guide clinical decisions. The literature on evidence-based medicine discusses the need to adopt a practice approach which turns clinical problems into questions, and then systematically locating, appraising and using the research findings to make informed clinical decisions. It has been estimated that for a doctor the process of formulating the question, finding the evidence, appraising it and acting on it can take about two hours, or longer if it is a complex problem.[8] There are concerns about the practicalities of adopting this approach, with many doctors and other health professionals commenting that there are already too few hours in the day to give patients the time they need and additionally cope with all of the paperwork.

Whilst there is a responsibility for individual professionals to provide care which is appropriate in the light of up-to-date evidence, most patient care is delivered by teams or by professionals working in collaboration. In such situations, evidence-based clinical practice is not the responsibility of each individual working in isolation, but is a team responsibility. Although such a specific approach as formulating the question, finding the evidence, appraising it and acting on it cannot be used by each practitioner for every single clinical encounter for every single patient, many clinical teams have decided to focus on specific clinical topics or areas as a starting point for assessing whether the care currently being given is based on the best evidence.

Although the reluctance of some health professionals to change past practice may result in care based on habit and opinion, there are also examples of new procedures or treatments being adopted by clinicians before adequate evaluation; for example laparoscopic cholecystectomy was rapidly introduced into the NHS and subsequent publications of a randomised controlled trial showed that there was little benefit associated with the procedure.[9] Healthcare practitioners also need to integrate the best evidence with their individual clinical expertise. Individual clinicians acquire proficiency and judgement through experience and practice, and the evidence may indicate a treatment or a procedure that a practitioner is not proficient in, and will need this to be shown or supervised before they can apply it. Clinical judgements may also be required to determine whether the best treatment for a particular condition is also the most suitable for a specific patient.

Yet how do healthcare practitioners find good research and evidence to guide their clinical decisions from the wealth of published healthcare information? And what is good research and evidence? Good evidence about a condition is an essential starting point for treating a patient with that condition, but no more than a starting point. The clinician then assesses whether local and patient-specific factors require the theoretically optimum treatment to be modified or rejected.

Evidence

A definition of evidence is 'something which provides ground for belief or disbelief'.[2] One of the first attempts to specify the strength of practice recommendations was in 1978 by the Canadian Task Force on the Periodic Health Examination.[10] However, this was not a very explicit framework as the evidence was only labelled as 'good', 'fair' or 'poor'. In 1992, the United States Department of Health and Human Services' Agency for Health Care Policy and Research identified levels and types of evidence, and this categorisation appears, or is referred to, in many publications relating to evidence-based care.[11] These levels are:

Level	Type of evidence
Ia	Evidence obtained from meta-analysis of randomised controlled trials
Ib	Evidence obtained from at least one randomised controlled trial
IIa	Evidence obtained from at least one well-designed controlled study without randomisation
IIb	Evidence obtained from at least one other type of well-designed quasi-experimental study
III	Evidence obtained from well-designed non-experimental descriptive studies, such as comparative studies, correlation studies and case control studies
IV	Evidence obtained from expert committee reports or opinions and/or clinical experiences of respected authorities

Randomised controlled trials

Within medical research, the randomised controlled trial (RCT) is said to be the 'gold standard' when deciding whether a treatment is effective. RCTs provide the least biased estimation of the relative effects of alternative forms of treatment as large, random samples are used and every effort is made to minimise the possibility of error in design and conduct.

In medicine the importance of using RCTs has been recognised for some time and studies have been undertaken in many areas of medical diagnosis and treatment, with new drug therapies being a common treatment evaluated by RCT. There are, however, many areas of medicine in which RCTs are ethically undesirable and practically impossible.

Nurses are the largest professional workforce in the NHS and deliver most of the 'hands on' patient care. Although research in nursing has been undertaken since Florence Nightingale's studies, many nurses are likely to believe that there have been very few RCTs on the effectiveness of nursing practice. An appraisal study was undertaken to determine if RCTs have often been used to evaluate nursing, the study used both electronic databases and hand searching of nursing journals to find relevant articles, and this resulted in 522 reports of RCTs being identified.[12]

The professions allied to medicine (PAMs) have rarely been involved in randomised controlled trials – one reason being that there has been low funding for research into the interventions of PAMs, another being that the use of RCTs to evaluate the effectiveness of these interventions is not always the most ethical or appropriate method.

Meta-analysis

A meta-analysis of RCTs is an analysis of several RCTs on the same problem, but involves undertaking certain processes and techniques. Meta-analysis is 'a statistical synthesis of the numerical results of several trials that all examined the same question'.[13] The papers published on meta-analysis of RCTs may look daunting to many healthcare practitioners, and the immediate reaction may be 'I don't know enough about statistics to understand this'. However, a good meta-analysis can be easier for a non-statistician to understand than reading all of the original published research papers. The research trials may have been written up in different ways, but meta-analysis tabulates certain relevant information which means that the reader is able to compare the methodology and results of the trials. The original published papers may not have included all of the information the meta-analyst requires and so the authors of the trials will have been approached to request the raw data from which to calculate the required figures. Meta-analyses include trials that, on their own, did not demonstrate a significant difference between treatment and control; yet when the results of all the studies are combined there may be a result that is statistically significant. A well-known example of this is the meta-analysis of seven trials of the effect of administration of corticosteroids to mothers expected to give birth prematurely. Only two of the trials had shown a statistically significant benefit in relation to the survival of the infant, but the meta-analysis combined the results of the available studies and showed that infants of mothers treated with steroids were 30–50% less likely to die than infants of mothers in the control group.

There have been challenges to the use of meta-analyses as the basis for clinical practice. The main arguments have been that meta-analyses of RCTs only provide information at the population level and do not tell the practitioner about the causal processes in the individuals who compose the group. Group averages may also mask errors and inconsistencies. There is also concern that the narrow selection criteria used to recruit patients to trials (for example, many trials do not recruit patients who have more than one disease) means that there is limited applicability of the results to the general patient population (as many patients have more than one concurrent health problem).

Although meta-analyses of RCTs and individual RCTs, are at the top of the hierarchy of evidence, it needs to be remembered that the findings of a poorly undertaken study with methodological flaws should not be considered as providing better evidence than a large well-designed study from one of the lower levels of the hierarchy.

One of the frequently expressed concerns about evidence-based care is that it is restricted to RCTs and meta-analysis. One of the leading proponents of evidence-based medicine refutes that this is so and states that 'if no randomized controlled trial has been carried out for our patient's predicament, we follow the trail to the next best external evidence and work from there'.[14]

Quasi-experimental studies

The main difference between controlled studies and quasi-experimental studies is the lack of random assignment of the subjects to the experimental and control groups. There are many instances in healthcare evaluation where it is not possible to randomly assign people to an experimental and control group; for example, health visitors in one health authority may want to change an aspect of the way they work. The researchers may want to compare the outcomes of how things were before the change and how things were after the change had been implemented, and also compare the outcomes at the same points in time in a health authority where the changes have not occurred. In this situation there is no guarantee that the groups of people being compared in the two health authorities will be like each other. Apart from this the study design will be experimental with pre- and post-tests being conducted in both authorities.

Non-experimental studies

There are also instances where it is only possible to use non-experimental designs to undertake a study. Non-experimental designs cannot demonstrate causality, i.e. the studies cannot prove that A caused B. Therefore, findings from these studies are placed lower down in the hierarchy of evidence.

Expert committees and opinions

The lowest level of evidence is that obtained from expert committee reports, opinions or clinical experiences of respected authorities. All health professionals have a knowledge base of healthcare, but the facts and experiences gained during practice, continuing education and reading will be influenced by an individual's values, beliefs and personal interests. Thus experts' knowledge of evidence will be influenced by their own beliefs and personal research interests and their knowledge is likely to be incomplete. Sackett noted that clinicians are likely to overestimate the effectiveness of interventions based upon their own clinical experiences,[15] and it has also been suggested that experts may give greater weight to findings that support their belief.[16] However, there is a limited amount of evidence available to assist with clinical decision making, especially in the fields of general practice and non–acute care, and the only information available is that from experts or the clinical experience of respected authorities.

Qualitative research

The hierarchy of evidence described does not include studies from the field of qualitative research. Qualitative research is frequently dismissed as methodologically inferior and lacking the scientific and statistical rigour of experimental methods.[17,18] Experimental research designs can demonstrate that causal relationships exist, but they cannot show how causal processes work; whereas the focus of qualitative research is on issues of process. The strength of quantitative research is its reliability, i.e. the same measurement should yield the same results time after time, and the strength of qualitative research is its validity. Validity is 'the degree to which the technique measures what it purports to measure'.[19] Qualitative researchers aim to 'study things in their natural setting, attempting to make sense of, or interpret, phenomena in terms of the meanings people bring to them'.[20] Wilson-Barnett[21] comments that 'with qualitative description, rigour and evidence are produced by following a pathway and ensuring all steps are traceable and reviewable'.

A qualitative approach is usually adopted when the purpose of the research is to explore, interpret or gain a deeper understanding of a particular issue, and this approach has been used many times within the fields of mental health, nursing and evaluation of health services. Frequently, a qualitative study will be undertaken in order to gain a better understanding of a situation and to begin to define a hypothesis for a further quantitative study.

When searching for information about best practice, nurses and the professions allied to medicine may find that qualitative studies have been undertaken, but no quantitative studies, and will need to make a judgement about the value of the findings. Each research approach has established assumptions, and health professionals will need to be familiar with the assumptions for qualitative research studies before a judgement can be made about the findings. A useful source on qualitative research is *Qualitative Research in Health Care* – the text also highlights the differences between the quantitative and qualitative approaches to research.[22]

It is now accepted that there is a role for both quantitative and qualitative research within evidence-based care. The Centre for Evidence-based Nursing is currently undertaking a qualitative research project which is exploring how nurses perceive and use evidence in decision making in clinical practice.[23]

Balancing the evidence

Sometimes more than one type of evidence is required for a clinician to determine whether an actual intervention will do more good than harm. Usually harmful side effects of a treatment occur much more infrequently than the beneficial effects. Randomised controlled trials tend to be designed to assess the effectiveness of a treatment and the design may not be powerful enough to detect any side effects that may occur. Cohort studies may also need to be undertaken to assess the safety of the intervention and the evidence from both studies used by clinicians to assess the balance between the harm and the good of the intervention.

There are also instances where the evidence that is available is contradictory. Clinicians then need to consider the information provided and decide how they are going to manage this.

Gaps in the evidence

It is highly unlikely that there will ever be scientific evidence for all aspects of healthcare, not only because of the limitations to research funding but also because there are areas of care in which it is practically impossible to undertake well-designed quantitative or qualitative studies. There are also areas of care where it will be ethically undesirable to undertake studies. Even in those areas that have been well researched, there are also going to be gaps on many aspects of care.

A recent remit for the Clinical Standards Advisory Group (CSAG) was:

> To advise on the impact on clinical standards of available evidence on clinical effectiveness . . . review, in a representative sample of Health Authorities and Boards, the extent to which such evidence is available in the NHS, and the effects that such evidence has on clinical practice; and consider factors that have led to, or prevented, the adoption of practices based on evidence of clinical effectiveness.[24]

It was decided to choose the management of a patient with stroke as the basis on which to conduct the research. Stroke care requires a multidisciplinary approach, covers all aspects of the NHS, is an important health problem and there is extensive research available on the topic. The study found that even though stroke has been particularly well researched, there are still gaps in the evidence on the organisation of care, the efficacy of nursing and rehabilitation, and the effectiveness in routine practice of most interventions. Evidence about a particular intervention may exist, but there is very little evidence which is relevant when individual aspects of the patient's condition are taken into account. For example, evidence exists that a foot drop splint helps people to walk, but there is no evidence as to whether a foot drop splint is effective when the patient has neglect of that limb, or if there is additional sensory loss. These individual aspects of the patient's condition need to be integrated into the clinical decision making on the most appropriate care for that patient.

Clinicians may express frustration at the shortfall of good quality evidence relating to the provision of care to patients, but even though the CSAG study identified large gaps in the evidence for stroke care, it also found many instances where health professionals were unaware of the available evidence for treating patients with stroke. This may only have related to a small proportion of the total care given to patients, but implementation of these interventions would increase the proportion of clinical services shown by evidence to be effective and help reduce the inequality of provision of care to patients throughout the NHS. Hence, the importance of health professionals being aware of the evidence which does exist and knowing how to find it – topics covered in the next chapter.

References

1 Smith R (1996) Information in practice. *British Medical Journal*. **313**: 1062–8.

2 *Collins Compact English Dictionary*. Third edition (1995) HarperCollins Publishers, Glasgow.

3 Urquart C and Hepworth J (1994) *The Value to Postgraduate and Continuing Medical Education of Information Supplied by NHS Library and Information Services*. Department of Information and Library Studies, Aberystwyth.

4 Marshall JG (1992) The impact of the hospital library on clinical decision making: the Rochester Study. *Bulletin of the Medical Library Association*. **80**(2): 169–78.

5 Smith R (1991) Where is the wisdom . . .? *British Medical Journal*. **303**: 798–9.

6 Ellis J, Mulligan I, Rowe J and Sackett DL (1995) Inpatient general medicine is evidence-based. *Lancet*. **346**: 407–10.

7 Dubinsky M and Ferguson JH (1990) Analysis of the National Institutes of Health Medicare Coverage Assessment. *International Journal of Technology Assessment in Health Care*. **6**: 480–8.

8 Rosenberg W and Donald A (1995) Evidence based medicine: an approach to clinical problem solving. *British Medical Journal*. **310**: 1122–6.

9 Majeed AW, Try G, Nicholl JP *et al.* (1996) Randomised, prospective single blind comparison of laparoscopic versus small incision cholecystectomy. *Lancet*. **347**: 989–94.

10 Canadian Task Force on the Periodic Health Examination (1979) The periodic health examination. *Canadian Medical Association Journal*. **121**: 1193–254.

11 US Department of Health and Human Services, Public Health Service, Agency for Health Care Policy and Research (1992) *Acute Pain Management: operative or medical procedures and trauma.*

Agency for Health Care Policy and Research Publications, Rockville, MD.

12 Cullum N (1997) Identification and analysis of randomised controlled trials in nursing: a preliminary study. *Quality in Health Care.* 6: 2–6.

13 Greenhalgh T (1997) *How to Read a Paper: the basics of evidence-based medicine.* BMJ Publishing Group, London.

14 Sackett DL, Richardson WS, Rosenberg W and Haynes RB (1997) *Evidence-based Medicine: how to practice & teach EBM.* Churchill Livingstone, Edinburgh.

15 Sackett DL (1986) Rules of evidence and clinical recommendations on the use of anti-thrombotic agents. *Chest.* 89 (Suppl 2): 2S–3S.

16 Oxman AD and Guyatt GH (1993) The science of reviewing research. *Annals of the New York Academy of Science.* 309: 648–51.

17 Mays N and Pope C (1995) Rigour and qualitative research. *British Medical Journal.* 311: 109–12.

18 Stanley L and Wise S (1993) *Breaking Out: feminist consciousness and feminist research.* Routledge, London.

19 Abbott P and Sapsford R (1998) *Research Methods for Nurses and the Caring Professions.* Second edition. Open University Press, Buckingham.

20 Denzin NK and Lincoln YS (eds) (1994) *Handbook of Qualitative Research.* Sage Publications, London.

21 Wilson-Barnett J (1998) Evidence for nursing practice: an overview. *NTresearch.* 3(1): 12–14.

22 Mays N and Pope C (eds) (1996) *Qualitative Research in Health Care.* BMJ Publishing Group, London.

23 Cullum N (1998) Clinical effectiveness in nursing. *NTresearch.* 3(1): 15–18.

24 Clinical Standards Advisory Group (1998) *Clinical Effectiveness: report on clinical effectiveness using stroke care as an example.* The Stationery Office, London.

4 Information sources and techniques

There is a vast array of information available on healthcare. Information is a wide term and includes textual and numerical data. Textual information includes books, journals, reports, statutes, circulars, policy instructions and letters. Numerical information comprises all items presented as numeric data, such as population data, statistic analyses, surveys, epidemiological reports and minimum data sets. The role of information in the provision of healthcare, and the need to improve the co-ordination and quality of NHS library and information resources, were the focus for a series of seminars during 1992 and 1993.[1] These seminars and subsequent activities highlighted the needs of NHS staff for new resources, new skills and new technology to handle the information which is available.

The role of librarians in medical, nursing, postgraduate and health service libraries has changed over the last decade. Librarians are a valuable resource to all health professionals and many are passing on to health professionals their skills in information seeking and retrieval, either via formal sessions during induction programmes and educational programmes, or on a one-to-one basis. Postgraduate libraries are being encouraged to become multiprofessional, which involves not just allowing other professions access to the resources but ensuring that the resources meet the information needs of the different professions.

There are a large number of information sources that are available when seeking information for evidence-based practice and these sources are increasing. This chapter will focus on a few of these sources.

Using published literature

The main source of textual evidence is the published literature, and with around 4000 healthcare journals published each month worldwide, a clinician is confronted by a wide range of journals during a visit to the library. There are many reasons why a health professional reads: to keep up-to-date; to track a research interest; to answer specific clinical questions. A rapid scan through recent issues of the main journals helps to keep a clinician informed of professional developments. If looking for answers to a particular clinical question or problem, usually related to the work situation, the clinician will find and read the studies published in the recent journals. These are likely to cite further relevant references which are found and read, which in turn identify other interesting references, and so the clinician may follow a considerable paper chase.

Reading for research involves seeking information about a defined topic in order to obtain a comprehensive view of the current state of knowledge, uncertainty and areas of ignorance on the topic. Attempting to find the available evidence about a particular aspect of care requires focused reading at the level of reading for research.

Selecting which journals to search is difficult, and to access all the journals and books would be extremely time consuming and very expensive. There are now numerous journals available that provide summaries of the articles published, for example: *ACP Journal Club*, *Evidence Based Medicine*, *Evidence Based Nursing* and *Bandolier*. The *Effective Health Care Bulletin* is produced by the NHS Centre for Reviews and Dissemination and the Nuffield Institute of Health, University of Leeds. Each bulletin focuses on a topic and consists of a systematic review and synthesis of research on the clinical effectiveness, cost effectiveness and acceptability of health service interventions. Stroke rehabilitation, the treatment of persistent glue ear in children, cholesterol (screening and treatment), and the prevention of pressure sores are just a few examples of the topics from the bulletins. *Effectiveness Matters* provides summaries of the clinical and cost effectiveness of particular healthcare interventions, and some examples of topics covered are aspirin and myocardial infarction, *Helicobacter pylori* and peptic ulcer and smoking cessation (what the health service can do).

Structuring literature enquiries

Health professionals seeking information in relation to clinical problems need to be clear about exactly what the question is to which they are seeking an answer. The clinician may have a problem in mind, but just looking through the journals and reading any articles on stroke will not help the searcher find the specific articles to answer directly the question 'will splinting prevent contractures occurring in this 68 year old woman who had a cerebrovascular accident 24 hours ago?'. Structuring the question will allow for efficient use of the searcher's time and enable a more precise answer to the clinical enquiry. Four components to a clinical question have been identified:[2]

1   the patient or problem
2   the intervention being considered
3   an alternative intervention which may include no intervention
4   the outcome.

Trying to find articles to answer the specific question just by randomly searching the journals will be very time consuming, as the question in this format may not be an area that has been covered in the summary journals and publications. Using electronic databases can speed up the process of finding relevant publications.

Electronic databases

Electronic bibliographic databases can help to save time in identifying the evidence; however, they can also provide an overwhelming amount of information, and not all of it is appropriate! As with reading there are approaches to using the electronic databases – either browsing and finding a lot of information of limited use, or conducting a systematic search. Again, having a clear question, such as 'will splinting prevent contractures occurring in this 68 year old woman who had a cerebrovascular accident 24 hours ago?', is the first step in the systematic search. For example, if the searcher just used the term 'stroke' then the database would find every reference relating to cerebrovascular stroke and heat stroke. The different types of electronic bibliographic databases make use of different search techniques and so slightly different strategies may need to be adopted. Before using any electronic database for the first time, it is recommended that a session is booked with a trained librarian or experienced user in order to understand the basics of the particular system.

The most well-known medical electronic bibliographic database is MedLine. This is a very large database of journal literature and is compiled by the National Library of Medicine of the United States. It covers the literature back to 1966, although not all of the journals currently indexed were included, or available, then. It does not contain the full article, usually only abstracts. Most medical and science libraries have access to MedLine, originally via telephone line connection into the main computer in the USA. The main computer can also be accessed over the Internet and other electronic services. Technological advances mean that the whole database is available in CD-ROM format, and many medical, nursing and postgraduate libraries have these and the required hardware to read them. There are several commercial vendors of the MedLine CD-ROM software, who may make use of different search techniques. The British Medical Association (BMA) library uses MedLine CD-ROMs and provides a dial-up service for all BMA members with a modem to access.

Undertaking a search using MedLine has become easier for clinicians with the advent of CD-ROM software, and references can be traced by any word listed on the database (these are words in the title, author's name, institution of author or where the research was undertaken, or a word in the abstract) or by use of a medical subject heading (MESH) term. Some of the CD-ROM software will automatically match the request to one of its standard MESH terms, other software will show the MESH terms if the 'suggest' button is clicked. When access was via telephone line connections to the mainframe computer in the USA, librarians tended to undertake the search on behalf of the clinician as the searcher needed to be skilled in the techniques and terms used in order to minimise the expensive connection charges. The basic skills can be learnt within a couple of hours, and the skills improved through use. For those clinicians who do not have access to a trained librarian or an experienced user, and may only have access to MedLine over the Internet, publications are now available which include some guidance on how to undertake a search.[3]

Having identified possible references the searcher may want to check whether the article does cover the required area of interest. The abstract of the article included in MedLine is the actual abstract that the author/s provided as part of the published literature; however, many nursing references identified by the search will not have an abstract as it is only recently that nursing journals have requested authors to include one. The abstract should provide an indication of the article's content to help the searcher decide whether there is a need to locate it. There may also be the introductory sentences of the article, but this may not be sufficient to indicate content, and the full article will need to be obtained.

Another major literature source is the Cumulative Index to Nursing and Allied Health Literature (CINAHL). This covers the English language literature related to nursing and the allied health disciplines and includes references from 1982 onwards. This database is a product of CINAHL Information Systems of California who index almost 700 journals.

Although electronic databases do provide access to references from a wide number of journals, it needs to be remembered that no one database provides access to all of the journals – hence, important articles can be missed if a search is undertaken using only one database. For example, MedLine does not index articles from the UK publication *Quality in Health Care*. There have been several studies comparing MedLine and CINAHL as there is considerable overlap between the coverage of nursing journals and therapist journals. Retrieval of the reference is dependent on the index terms used, and studies have shown that MedLine assigns more index terms to each article, but that CINAHL used index terms more focused on nursing topics.[4] Another study concluded that CINAHL was the preferred database for nursing students as it provided the higher percentage of relevant references and those of the greatest appropriateness, whilst a separate study concluded that both databases were valuable for the professions allied to medicine.[5,6] Although there are different emphases by the study authors, a common conclusion was that both MedLine and CINAHL should be used for comprehensive searches.

Use of electronic bibliographic databases does not guarantee finding all of the evidence available. It takes time for articles to be indexed, and CD-ROM software has to be updated, usually quarterly, to ensure that new publications are included. Not all relevant articles entered onto the bibliographic databases may be retrieved during a search. The selection by authors, editors and indexers of key words for indexing may not be the most appropriate for a specific retrieval, and the grouping of articles under subheadings and types in abstracts is also open to human error. It has been estimated that about half of the material listed on MedLine can only be accessed in a specific context by looking through the journals again. It has also been identified that of the randomised controlled trials in MedLine, approximately half will be found by an expert searcher, and only half of these will be found by an experienced clinical user.[7] One way of overcoming the difficulties of identifying randomised controlled trials is by using the Cochrane Library. Finally, to overcome the effects of inevitable time lags, even if the search to answer the clinical question is being conducted on the latest database update there will still be a need to hand search journals, especially the latest numbers.

The Cochrane Library

Originally named the Cochrane Database of Systematic Reviews when launched in 1995, the Cochrane Library contains:

- the Cochrane Database of Systematic Reviews (CDSR)
- the York Database of Abstracts of Reviews of Effectiveness (DARE)
- the Cochrane Controlled Trials Register (CCTR)
- the Cochrane Review Methodology Database (CRMD).

The electronic library is the result of the Cochrane Collaboration's work in uncovering and reviewing high quality research evidence. The Cochrane Collaboration is an international network of health professionals, researchers and consumers and has two main types of organisational units: Cochrane Centres and Collaborative Review Groups. The Collaboration has developed an efficient search strategy for MedLine, and is working with the National Library of Medicine to improve the identification of both old and newly published trials through MedLine. In addition, there is hand searching of journals. Reviewers prepare specific protocols for each review undertaken, and software developed by the Collaboration provides an organisational and analytical framework for assembling the reviews. There is a rapidly growing collection of information about high level evidence, but this is not yet comprehensive as the systematic processes used to identify and review the information take time. Therefore, the area of clinical care that a clinician is specifically interested in seeking evidence on may not yet be included. Many medical and postgraduate libraries subscribe to the Cochrane Library which is frequently used first to identify any randomised controlled trials or other high level evidence.

NHS Centre for Reviews and Dissemination

The health departments of England, Wales, Scotland and Northern Ireland fund the NHS Centre for Reviews and Dissemination (CRD). The Centre provides the Database of Abstracts of Reviews of Effectiveness (DARE), which is available on the Cochrane Library disk and the NHS Economic Evaluation Database. DARE is a set of records of reviews of the effectiveness of healthcare interventions and the organisation of healthcare delivery published since 1994. The trained reviewers and information staff from CRD carefully evaluate, against a set of criteria, the reports from the world literature and provide a structured abstract which includes the aims and main findings, and a critical appraisal of the methods used. The NHS Economic Evaluations Database (NEED) contains detailed abstracts which summarise and critically appraise individual reports of economic evaluations of healthcare.

Practicalities of using electronic databases

Clinicians are making more use of electronic bibliographic databases and many libraries now operate a booking system. Librarians still provide an information seeking and retrieval service and may block out time in the day during which only they have access to the databases. Prior checking for availability of the database for a particular time may, therefore, be an advantage.

Having obtained the relevant references from the database, the searcher then needs to locate the actual articles and read these. Some of the publications will be held in the local library, but some may not. Nowadays, there is better sharing of information among local or regional libraries, with each library knowing which publications others hold, and requests between libraries for photocopies of articles are common. However, some more specialist articles may have to be requested from the British Library by the local librarian. The Copyright Licensing Agency identifies the rules relating to the photocopying of copyright material (namely published material). These rules are upheld and any infingement of them is a serious offence. Libraries and other institutions must hold a licence before any photocopying is undertaken and exactly what, and how many, can be copied will depend on the type of licence held. For example, a basic licence does not include an agreement for any copying of course pack copyright material. The person requesting the article has to complete and sign a form regardless of the library approached. This inter-library loan form contains statements relating to the copyright licence, and the form is explicit in making clear that the copy requested should only be used for research or private study and the requester should not supply a copy to any other person. This should be remembered – any article obtained cannot be copied for everyone else within the clinical team.

The photocopying services of libraries vary – many make a charge for any photocopying while others provide a free service for work use and a charge for personal use. Some libraries make a charge to the user for photocopies obtained from other libraries, or they may be funded from each department based on a departmental estimation of usage of the library services. Which ever system is used the photocopying costs within libraries have increased as more clinicians are seeking information on which to base their practice. There may also be significant delays in obtaining either copies of articles or the actual publication or book itself, as more and more requests are made. If health organisations want to support evidence-based practice, they need to acknowledge the likely costs generated by accessing and retrieving the information needed to make decisions about the effectiveness of care.

Internet

Although there have been improvements in the availability of library facilities, it has not been universal. Many libraries have restricted opening or are several miles away for staff working in the community or smaller hospitals. Even when on the same site clinicians may still not find it easy to visit due to the demands of their clinical duties. However, numerous people have personal access to the Internet and this may be the information source used by many health professionals. The Internet provides several millions of pages of information and many will contain information about health; however, it should be remembered that there is no quality control over the information available. To help filter out unsuitable or out of date information, the Organising Medical Networked Information (OMNI) project was started as an Electronic Libraries Programme. All resources entered into OMNI have been assessed for quality and are reviewed regularly. The items are indexed to improve retrieval, classified for easy browsing and have a short description attached to allow the searcher to decide in advance whether a resource will provide the information required. Resources are also divided into two groups, UK and worldwide.

As previously mentioned, MedLine is available on the Internet and there is access to journals such as *ACP Journal Club* and *Bandolier*. A good starting point for information and lists of Internet resources which support clinical effectiveness and evidence-based practice is *Netting the Evidence: a ScHARR introduction to evidence-based practice on the internet.* (*http://www.shef.ac.uk/uni/academic/R-Z/scharr/ir/netting.html*).

Health professionals in Wales identified that they needed access to high quality information, the skills to find and use that information and an environment which supported clinical effectiveness. One aspect of the clinical effectiveness initiative was to investigate new methods of information dissemination. Wales established its own private intranet – NHS CymruWeb – consisting of a number of web servers built and maintained by health authorities, trusts and other organisations throughout Wales. It offers easy access to information, services, resources and communications facilities and the Cymru-Web facilities include healthcare bibliographic databases such as MedLine and CINAHL, official documents, newsletters, news groups and e-mail. The New Information for Clinical Effectiveness (NICE) project was established, its aim to ensure that a significant number of health professionals were able to use on-line sources of healthcare information for practice by co-ordinating access, providing skills training and providing on-going support. The training does not just teach users how to access NHS CymruWeb successfully, but also how to define the clinical problem, devise a search strategy, retrieve relevant information and develop critical appraisal skills. By the end of 1998, NICE enabled over 200 multidisciplinary teams from a range of settings (health authority, acute trusts, community trusts, general practice, dental practice) to have access to, training in and help-desk, help-line support for this information. The project also used a variety of techniques to evaluate the service.

If you are not familiar with using the Internet there are books available to help, including one in this health informatics series.[8]

The grey literature

The term 'grey literature' covers an informal but well understood category of reports, circulars, letters and documents not published in the conventional way. Not all researchers write an article for the scientific press, and, for a variety of reasons, not every article submitted is published. For a long time qualitative research studies were considered to be of little importance and articles were not published in the leading journals – journals also tended not to print research articles which showed no or little results. These academic research reports may be of relevance. Other documents in this category include locally produced documents such as needs assessment reports, working papers, theses and dissertations, statistical reports, strategy documents and policy statements.

It is also important to identify research in progress. The four UK countries maintain a register of research that the respective R&D programmes are funding (*see* Chapter 2) and there is also a database of US government and private foundation funded current health services research.

Finding and obtaining the information can be time consuming, not simply in the actual time it takes to undertake the searches, but in waiting for the publications to arrive if they are not held in the local library. This can be frustrating for the healthcare team anxious to improve their care and there is a temptation to use just the information available from the local sources. All of the information is required before a decision can be made about the appropriateness of care. However, while waiting the available articles can be read and appraised. The next chapter discusses how to appraise the information.

References

1 Haines M (1995) The Cumberlege Seminars in England. *Health Informatics.* 1: 3–9.
2 Sackett DL, Richardson WS, Rosenberg WS and Haynes RB (1997) *Evidence-based Medicine: how to practice & teach EBM.* Churchill Livingstone, Edinburgh.
3 Greenhalgh T (1997) *How to Read a Paper: the basics of evidence-based medicine.* BMJ Publishing Group, London.
4 Brenner SH and McKinin EJ (1989) CINAHL and MedLine: a comparison of indexing practices. *Bulletin of the Medical Library Association.* 77: 366–71.

5   Okuma E (1994) Selecting CD-ROM databases for nursing students: a comparison of MedLine and the Cumulative Index to Nursing and Allied Health Literature (CINAHL). *Bulletin of the Medical Library Association.* **82**: 25–9.

6   Watson MM and Perrin R (1994) A comparison of CINAHL and McdLine CD-ROM in four allied health areas. *Bulletin of the Medical Library Association.* **82**: 214–16.

7   Adams CE, Power A, Frederick K and Lefebvre C (1994) An investigation of the adequacy of MedLine searches for randomized controlled trials (RCTs) of the effect of mental health care. *Psychological Medicine.* **24**: 741–8.

8   Tyrrell S (1999) *Using the Internet in Healthcare.* Radcliffe Medical Press, Oxford.

5 Appraising the information

Once apparently relevant articles have been identified, they need to be read to determine whether the evidence is valid (means what it claims to mean), useful (includes important findings) and appropriate for the local situation (relevant). Many journals send out papers received to referees for comments on the clarity of writing and the paper's scientific validity, originality and importance. (The journal's instructions to authors usually states whether some or all of the papers received are sent out for peer review.) A reader might assume that if articles have been peer reviewed then the evidence presented is suitable to use to inform practice; however, this is not the case and all research papers should be subject to critical appraisal. Although many health professionals will say that they do this all of the time, there are also many who realise that they may need to have a more informed understanding of how to appraise critically a research paper. Using a logical framework which is structured around questions that enable the reader to determine whether a paper is valid, useful and relevant means that a reasoned judgement about the paper can be reached.

Developing critical appraisal skills

The literature on evidence-based medicine and evidence-based practice covers, in detail, structured guides on how to read papers on diagnosis, screening, prognosis, therapy, economic analysis, systematic reviews, overviews, qualitative research and guidelines. *How to Read a Paper: the basis of evidence-based medicine* and *The Pocket Guide to Critical Appraisal* are likely to be found in many postgraduate libraries.[1,2] Basic education programmes for health professionals now provide critical appraisal skills training, as do many postgraduate training programmes. The postgraduate courses may use specially prepared workbooks such as *Practising Evidence-based Medicine* or open learning material such as *Evidence-based Primary Care*, both of which provide tutor information to enable the tutor to facilitate the sessions.[3,4] There are also training programmes that specifically teach critical appraisal skills and these may be half-day, two or three day, or week long courses. The shorter courses aim to promote an understanding of the nature of the evidence and the issues that need to be taken into account in judging the value of the evidence. These are not courses in statistics and are not intended to enable everyone to read every paper. Even when they have attended more intensive courses, most healthcare professionals still refer to a printed checklist of specific questions when critically appraising a research paper.

The aspects of critical appraisal that many practitioners express lack of confidence in are statistics and research design and methods, even if they have attended courses on these topics. Health practitioners are not experts in all areas of clinical care, and if a patient presents with problems that are outside their usual domain they seek advice from someone who is more experienced in that field. Similarly, health practitioners are not expected to be able to appraise comprehensively every single research paper that they read. Advice may need to be sought from someone else within the clinical team who has more experience in a particular clinical area, or support obtained in a particular statistical technique from someone else in the organisation who has the necessary skills.

Several journals now publish original research papers plus a review of the paper, for example *Clinical Effectiveness for Nurses*, *NTresearch*. By using this approach the journals not only help with the dissemination of research, but also provide an environment for authors to develop their research and writing skills. These journals are also helpful to practitioners wanting to improve their critical appraisal skills as they can read and appraise the original research paper and then read the review of the paper and compare their comments to those made by the reviewer.

Whilst there is a responsibility for individual professionals to provide care which is appropriate in the light of up-to-date evidence, most patient care is delivered by teams or by professionals working in collaboration. In such situations, evidence-based clinical practice is not the responsibility of each individual working in isolation, but a team responsibility. Although individual members of the team may have been tasked with searching for relevant articles on which to review practice, it is frequently the team which critically appraises the articles found. Within the team there may be individuals who have the required knowledge to address all of the questions required for the critical appraisal of all the evidence located – if not, then people with these skills will need to be identified.

Key elements of critical appraisal

As previously mentioned there are many articles and books describing critical appraisal, providing structured guides for reviewing specific types of papers. These publications also highlight certain questions that ought to be considered for any paper. The next section presents the key points that these publications have identified as common factors for consideration regardless of the type of research paper being appraised.

There is a standard format that research papers are expected to follow, whether written up as a small project undertaken as part of a training programme, as a dissertation, or as a paper for a scientific journal. This is **Introduction; Methods; Results; Discussion**.

Introduction

The background to the study needs to define the topic or field, include a review of previous work, highlight the gaps in the knowledge, and explain why this particular study was carried out. Ideally, the final part should be a clear statement of the purpose of the study.

Methods

This is the most important section to look at to decide whether a paper is worth reading. It should contain sufficient information to indicate exactly who or what was studied, what type of study was undertaken and what methods were used in the collection and analysis of the data.

Detailed checklists produced for the critical appraisal of a paper are usually specific to a particular research method – there is therefore a need to identify first the research method being used for the study, remembering the levels and types of evidence discussed in Chapter 3. The reader then needs to decide whether this was the right type of study to examine the particular research question or topic. It may be helpful to have a book to hand which identifies either the basic research methods or the preferred methods for studies concerned with therapy, diagnosis, screening etc. The publication *How to Read a Paper: the basics of evidence-based medicine* highlights preferred study designs and describes the main research methods.[1]

Sufficient information should be provided to indicate who was studied and how they were recruited. This information is required in order to decide how widely the findings can be generalised and whether this information could be applicable to a specific set of patients. For example, the study may have been conducted on people from an ethnic group different from that of most local patients. There is also a need to know who was excluded from the study – for example, many trials exclude patients who have more than the one illness or condition being studied whereas patients presenting locally may have several coexisting illnesses including the one being studied. The section should also provide sufficient details about how the research subjects were recruited, what the actual sample size was, and whether any people withdrew or did not continue with the study.

The methods section needs to contain sufficient information to decide whether the data collected are likely to be accurate – for example, if a questionnaire was used had it been tested for validity and reliability prior to the main data collection? An indication of the statistical methods used in the analysis is also required.

The detailed checklists published assist the reader to undertake a more detailed appraisal of papers. Usually there are some standard questions which act as an initial filter to sift out papers with any major defects in the research. The rest of the checklist is divided into sections corresponding to the main sections of a research paper, and the more detailed questions in the method section will assist with assessing the overall quality of the study.

Results

This section should take the reader through the data and highlight the key findings. The results ought to be presented in a logical order, starting with the simple observations and finishing with any complex analyses. The results should address the aim of the study. Tables or graphs are frequently used and should be explained. At one time it was usual for papers to just present tables and graphs and an explanation of the main findings; now, a paper is expected to assess the statistical significance of the findings.

The majority of health professionals do not need to perform the various statistical tests themselves, but will need to know which statistical test is the best to use for common problems. Once again, having a book to hand that clearly describes the various basic statistical tests and their uses can be helpful.[5–8] If a study has used a test that is not in a basic statistics textbook, the author ought to clearly state why that test has been used and provide a reference which defines the test and its uses. The questions provided in the detailed checklists for specific research papers frequently include questions about the statistical tests that should have been undertaken as part of the study. Whilst statistics can often appear intimidating, the use of checklists means that most practitioners should be able to assess the statistical tests used in most healthcare research papers. If understanding of the finer points of statistical tests is required, then it is best to seek help from an expert.

Discussion

The wider implications of the study should be addressed in the discussion, and the findings should be compared with other studies undertaken. This section will need to be read with care to determine whether the authors have been impartial when interpreting the results and significance of their study.

The answers to the questions within the detailed critical appraisal of the paper should allow the reviewer, either an individual practitioner or the clinical team, to make a reasoned judgement about the validity, usefulness and appropriateness of the evidence. It is useful to make a summary of the information from the critical appraisal of the research papers − this helps in checking that all the relevant questions have been considered and highlights whether there are any differences in the evidence provided in the different papers.

When a clinical team is reviewing practice, it is likely that several members of the team have been asked to appraise critically the research papers and to bring their completed checklists and summary of information to a meeting involving all, or most, of the team. It is unusual for every research paper to present all of the required information in a format that is easily understood by every single person. Even using a structured approach, different team members may have identified slightly different aspects within the paper depending on their background and experience. Having a group of diverse people to critically review papers is useful and the discussion that ensues may help to clarify an individual's thoughts on an article, or make them think again about what they have noted. Many courses recommend that critical appraisal should be under-taken by a group of people with different knowledge and experi-ences. The discussion within the group also helps the group reach a consensus on the value of the evidence and whether there is a need to change practice.

If all of the evidence points in the same direction, it is usually prudent to follow it providing the reader has mapped the evidence to the local situation; however, there may not be a perfect answer from the evidence sources or the evidence may be conflicting or unclear. What needs to be remembered is that the evidence is intended to help determine best practice, and that the responsibility remains with the individual health professional and the test for 'reasonableness', with the evidence being the guide as to what is 'reasonable' under the circumstances.

References

1   Greenhalgh T (1997) *How to Read a Paper: the basics of evidence-based medicine*. BMJ Publishing Group, London.
2   Crombie IM (1996) *The Pocket Guide to Critical Appraisal*. BMJ Publishing Group, London.
3   Straus SE, Badenoch D, Richardson WS *et al.* (1998) *Practising Evidence-based Medicine*. Radcliffe Medical Press, Oxford.
4   Carter Y and Falshaw M (eds) (1998) *Evidence-based Primary Care. Workbooks 1–6*. Radcliffe Medical Press, Oxford.
5   Bradford Hill A and Hill ID (1991) *Principles of Medical Statistics* (12th ed). Arnold, London.
6   Armitage P and Berry G (1994) *Statistical Methods in Medical Research* (3rd ed). Blackwell, Oxford.
7   Bland M (1987) *An Introduction to Medical Statistics*. Oxford Medical Press, Oxford.
8   Jordan K, Ong BM and Croft P (1998) *Mastering Statistics: a guide for health service professionals and researchers*. Stanley Thornes, Cheltenham.

6 Clinical guidelines

Clinical decisions should be based on the best possible evidence of effectiveness. The increase in information has led to an increase in the complexity of decision making and clinicians are faced with the difficulty of finding the time to track down, collect and critically appraise research findings. Carefully evaluated summaries of available evidence are one mechanism which may assist healthcare professionals to keep abreast of new developments. The *Effective Health Care* bulletins (discussed in Chapter 4) are one example of evaluated summaries of available evidence, and clinical guidelines are another example.

Guidelines, protocols, profiles of care, clinical algorithms, standards and care plans were terms that the Scottish Clinical Resource and Audit Group found to be in use and were often treated as synonymous. The group recommended that 'the term "clinical guideline" should apply to the general statement of principle and the word "protocol" should cover the more detailed development of these broad principles for local application'.[1] However, this distinction does not appear to have been adopted throughout the UK, instead the phrases 'national guidelines' and 'local guidelines' are used. Recent literature appears to have adopted the term 'clinical guideline', with the preferred definition as 'systematically developed statements to assist practitioner and patient decisions about appropriate healthcare for specific clinical circumstances'.[2]

There has been much debate on the subject of clinical guidelines. One view is that guidelines are useful and clinicians want to use them to improve, and audit, the quality of healthcare they provide; whilst the opposite view is that as no two patients, or their illness, are identical then clinical guidelines take away the flexibility of matching care to individual patient need and inhibit innovation of practice. Another argument is that a patient's confidence in the practitioner may be reduced if the patient knows that guidelines are being used; however, the proposers highlight that many patients are aware that there is a wide variation in practice, and the knowledge that the practitioner is using agreed, up-to-date treatment is more likely to give the patient confidence.

Health departments are perceived, by some, to be driving the use of guidelines to reduce costs.[3] In England, purchasers have been encouraged to include evidence-based guidelines in their contracts as a method of increasing clinical effectiveness. Within Scotland and Wales, the use of guidelines has been encouraged to improve patient care and reduce variation in practice, and it has been acknowledged that, occasionally, optimal practice may be more expensive than current practice. It has also been identified that investment is required for the development and implementation of clinical guidelines, but that 'this investment should be accepted as a method of improving patient care rather than as a means of cost cutting'.[1]

It has been shown that valid guidelines, appropriately disseminated and implemented, are capable of producing beneficial changes in clinical practice and improvements in patient outcomes.[4] However, the 'dissemination and implementation of invalid guidelines may lead to wasteful use of resources on ineffective interventions or, even worse, deterioration in patients' health'.[5]

Appraisal of clinical guidelines

There has been a proliferation of guidelines available for clinicians to use, yet clinicians need to reassure themselves that each guideline will achieve its intended outcome of improving practice and improving patient outcomes. The first step in this is appraisal of the quality of the guideline. The literature has discussed the desirable attributes of clinical practice guidelines and, more recently, an *Appraisal Instrument for Clinical Guidelines* has been published which takes into account the initial work undertaken in both the United Kingdom and the USA.[6] The appraisal instrument is intended for independent assessment of existing guidelines and for use as an aide memoir by guideline developers. Rigour of development, context and content, and application of the guideline are the three dimensions of the appraisal instrument. There is also a user guide which is intended to ensure that the questions within the three sections are interpreted consistently.

Guideline development

How, and by whom, guidelines are developed can affect their potential use. As with all evidence-based practice, guidelines should be based on the best available evidence. This means that a systematic approach to identifying, synthesising and interpreting evidence needs to take place with an explicit link between the major recommendations and the level of supporting evidence. Unfortunately, many guidelines have been developed by 'expert' groups who have relied on their own knowledge of published work, rather than a systematic review of the literature using established techniques. The strength of the evidence in the different areas of the guideline needs to be evaluated, and there are likely to be some areas where rigorous evidence is lacking. The task of interpreting the evidence to inform guideline recommendation is not easy and a group also needs to assess the relevance of the studies identified to the target population of the guideline. Most guideline documentation will contain a mixture of evidence-linked and consensus-based recommendations. It is crucial that the areas of clinical uncertainty are clearly identified, and it has been suggested that those interventions where there is a lack of evidence on their effectiveness are presented as options within the guideline.[7]

Currently, guidelines originate from a wide variety of organisations and England's NHS Executive has highlighted criteria to use for guideline selection – only those guidelines based upon randomised controlled trials, and expert opinion that has been endorsed by 'respected authorities' would be considered for commendation.[8] Approved guidelines only account for a very small proportion of the total number of guidelines in circulation, so health professionals need to remember to review guidelines before using them to guide practice.

It is recommended that a multidisciplinary process should be used to develop guidelines and the various professional bodies and organisations (medical, nursing and professions allied to medicine) are involved with the development of guidelines.[9] However, there are very few multiprofessional guidelines currently available, and guidelines development has tended to be 'uni-professional' with limited use of other professionals. Many guidelines are often a description of the medical, nursing or professions allied to medicine management of a particular condition rather than the overall care of patients with that particular condition. An essential component for a multiprofessional clinical guideline is clarity of each profession's role and responsibility for appropriate care; true multiprofessional team working is still evolving and there is a large learning curve for all professional groups to work together at both national and local level.

Another practical issue relating to the development of multi-disciplinary guidelines is the potential size of the group to achieve the balance of all interested disciplines. If the group is too large it may be difficult to lead and achieve cohesiveness. It is suggested that the optimum size for a small group is between six and ten people,[10] yet for most guideline development groups this is not sufficient to represent all interests and a larger-than-optimum group will be needed. The group requires a leader skilled in small-group leadership who can ensure that the group is not dominated by a minority of its members and that all members make a contribution. The initial step for the group not only includes defining the task, but also developing a mutual respect for, and understanding of, different professionals' experiences, and developing a method for dealing with conflict.

Developing and applying national guidelines

Skills and considerable resources are required to develop valid guidelines. The Scottish Clinical Resource and Audit Group suggested that national resources should be used to develop valid guidelines which can be adapted to local resources and circumstances, and the Scottish Intercollegiate Guidelines Network (SIGN) was given responsibility for sponsoring and appraising national guidelines and co-ordinating activity to prevent duplication of effort.[1] The recent English and Welsh White Papers on the new NHS recommend that guidelines be produced and disseminated via the National Institute of Clinical Excellence (NICE).[11,12] NICE is intended to reduce duplication of activity and maximise the use of professional and academic expertise needed to produce credible guidelines.

The Royal College of General Practitioners has suggested that the first steps are the local adaptation of national (or regional) valid guidelines.[13] This approach means that at a national level skills and expertise in conducting systematic reviews, synthesising evidence, and developing valid guidelines are required. Skills in the appraisal and adaptation of national guidelines are required locally, as well as the ability to identify local resource constraints and barriers to implementation. This local guideline development group should be representative of the professional groups, and include managers who are required to support the successful implementation of the guideline and the monitoring of its use, including whether it has achieved the expected outcomes. The local guideline group needs to remember that the actual number of guidelines that a health professional or an organisation can assimilate at any time is limited, and should consider the local situation when determining which national guidelines to adapt for local use.

Consumer involvement in guidelines

The focus of guidelines is clinical practice and patients and consumers need to become integral in the process of guideline development and review. Currently, there is little evidence of active involvement of consumers in guideline development groups. The role of consumers within evidence-based practice is discussed in Chapter 7.

Style and format of guidelines

Guidelines have a wide range of styles and formats and there is little information available on the effect that these have on guideline adoption. Clarity is important – of definitions, language and format – to ensure that different users interpret and apply the guideline in the same way. Clinical terms need to be used precisely, and statements need to be unambiguous. Whatever the format there needs to be sufficient documentation to identify the participants of the guideline development group; the procedures and methods used in the guideline development; the strengths of the evidence, assumptions and rationales used; and the method of peer review of the guideline. Most guidelines contain insufficient documentation for potential users to appraise adequately the guidelines' validity and relevance to specific circumstances. The guideline documentation should identify outcomes for monitoring as well as an indication of how it should be reviewed to incorporate any major changes in knowledge.

Medico-legal concerns

There have been, and continue to be, concerns from many clinicians about the medico-legal issues around guidelines. Practitioners ask whether clinical guidelines will be used to decide whether the care they provided was substandard, or whether they will be considered negligent because they have not followed a particular guideline, even though the NHSE publication stated that guidelines are to assist the practitioner and they '. . . cannot be used to mandate, authorise or outlaw treatment options . . .'[8] Articles have been published relating to these concerns and a useful publication *Clinical Guidelines and the Law* clarifies the legal status of guidelines, the legal liability of guideline writers and includes summaries of key legal cases and key articles on the legal significance of guidelines.[14] The book also includes selected further reading, providing not only the author, title and source, but a brief resume of the article.

Dissemination and implementation of guidelines

Having a valid clinical guideline is just the first step towards its successful adoption. The guideline needs to be actively disseminated to relevant clinicians with strategies aimed at influencing clinicians' awareness, attitudes, knowledge and understanding of the guideline. Implementation strategies encouraging clinicians to change their clinical practice in line with the guideline are also needed. There have been studies conducted into the role of operational clinical support systems and guideline uptake. Patient-specific reminders and alerts based on given circumstances appeared to be a factor in the likelihood of guideline effectiveness; however, there are still very few UK healthcare organisations that can provide this type of support.[15]

Whilst publication of the guideline in professional journals, or mailing to relevant groups, can influence healthcare professionals' awareness of the guideline, more active participation via targeted seminars, educational programmes or the use of opinion leaders may be more likely to change behaviour. Although there have been some studies comparing different strategies, further research is still needed to identify those most likely to be successful in different contexts.

There is a danger that the proliferation of guidelines may defeat their purpose as 'systematically developed statements to assist practitioner and patient decisions about appropriate healthcare for specific clinical circumstances'.[2] A survey of guidelines in general practice, in one particular health authority, identified 855 different guidelines, with a massive increase of guidelines production since 1989.[16] Clinicians need information to be easily accessible and usable so that they can use it at the point of care or contact. Use of the electronic medium needs to be explored more in order for clinicians to be able to search for relevant guidelines and to have updated, not old, versions of guidelines.

References

1   Clinical Resource and Audit Group (1993) *Clinical Guidelines: Report of a working group.* Scottish Office Home and Health Department, Edinburgh.

2   Institute of Medicine (Field MJ and Lohr KN eds) (1992) *Guidelines for Clinical Practice: from development to use.* National Academy Press, Washington DC.

3   Newton J, Knight D and Woolhead G (1996) General practitioners and clinical guidelines: a survey of knowledge, use and beliefs. *British Journal of General Practice.* **46**: 513–17.

4   Effective Health Care (1994) *Implementing Clinical Practice Guidelines: can guidelines be used to improve clinical practice?* Bulletin No. 8. University of Leeds, Leeds.

5   Grimshaw J, Eccles M and Russell I (1995) Developing clinically valid practice guidelines. *Journal of Evaluation in Clinical Practice.* **1**: 37–48.

6   Cluzeau F, Littlejohns P, Grimshaw J and Feder G (1997) *Appraisal Instrument for Clinical Guidelines.* St George's Hospital Medical School, London.

7   Eddy DM (1992) *A Manual for Assessing Health Practices and Designing Practice Policies: the explicit approach.* American College of Physicians, Philadelphia.

8   NHS Executive (1996) *Clinical guidelines: using clinical guidelines to improve patient care within the NHS.* Department of Health, Leeds.

9   Grimshaw JM and Russell IT (1993) Achieving health gain through clinical guidelines I: developing scientifically valid guidelines. *Quality in Health Care.* **2**: 243–8.

10 Øvretveit J (1993) *Coordinating Community Care.* Open University Press, Buckingham.

11 Secretary of State (1997) *A First Class Service: quality in the new NHS.* Cmnd 3807. HMSO, London.

12 Welsh Office (1998) *Quality Care and Clinical Excellence.* Welsh Office, Cardiff.

13 Royal College of General Practitioners (1995) *The Development and Implementation of Clinical Guidelines: Report of the Clinical Guidelines Working Group.* Report from Practice 26. Royal College of General Practitioners, London.

14 Hurwitz B (1998) *Clinical Guidelines and the Law: negligence, discretion and judgment.* Radcliffe Medical Press, Oxford.

15 Johnston ME, Langton KB, Haynes RB and Mathieu A (1994) Effects

of computer-based clinical decision support systems on clinician performance and patient outcome: a critical appraisal of research. *Annals of Internal Medicine.* **120**: 135–42.

16   Hibble A, Kanka D, Pencheon D and Pooles F (1998) Guidelines in general practice: the new Tower of Babel? *British Medical Journal.* **317**: 862–3.

7 Patient information

Health information leaflets and booklets can be found in the waiting areas of GP surgeries, in outpatient departments, within hospital wards, in chemist shops, public libraries and many other public places. The availability and accessibility of health information to the public within the UK, has increased significantly since the 1980s. This has been in response to the increasing demands for health and other information by society and government policies which have placed greater importance on consumer choice, including the provision of health information to patients.[1,2] A study undertaken in 1987 found that information on specific diseases and medical conditions were the main areas in which people required health information.[3] This information was wanted not only as a source of reassurance, but also to enable individuals to participate in their own care or that of a relative. Group interviews undertaken as part of this study identified that people felt that health professionals provided too little information, and that information was unlikely to be volunteered unless the patient asked questions. In 1993, an Audit Commission report also identified that patients did not get all of the information that they wanted or needed.[4]

Within the UK there is very limited choice, i.e. alternatives, for healthcare as the NHS is the main provider of health services. There has been an increased emphasis on patient participation and the clinical effectiveness initiatives have highlighted the need for health professionals and managers to work in partnership with patients – but what does this actually mean?[5,6] There is an increasing volume of literature relating to 'patient participation', however there appears to be a lack of clarity in the terminology and underlying concepts which makes it difficult to make comparisons or form any conclusions. 'Choice', 'involvement', 'collaboration' and 'empowerment' are terms that appear to be used interchangeably, and there also appears to be confusion between the process of giving and receiving information and 'participation' in decision making.

Decision making

It has been suggested that the main point of giving patients information is to help them reach a decision[7] and that patients want information to reduce anxiety and combat fear,[8,9] and to make it easier to comply with, or reject, clinical decisions.[10] Several authors have also highlighted that wanting information is not the same as wanting to be in charge.[9,11,12] Hope has highlighted that having information is not sufficient for patients to exercise choice:

> . . . to exercise choice patients need to have power to choose . . .
> Patients need to be genuinely involved in the process of making
> healthcare decisions.[7]

Decision making is concerned with making choices between alternative options and weighing the benefits and risks. Traditionally, the clinicians' preferences, expert knowledge and values have been used to make decisions with which patients are expected to comply; however, this approach does not recognise that patients have their own perceptions, values and preferences. It also needs to be remembered that, under English law, a competent person has a right to accept or refuse the treatment (even life-saving) on offer.[7] In order to make this choice the patient requires the relevant information.

There is increasing evidence about the benefits of giving information to patients, but there is little agreement about how involved patients want to be in the clinical decision making process.[13] The study by Deber et al. of patients with heart disease found that there were relatively high levels of desire for information and a wish to be involved in decision making, but a strong desire for doctors to make technical treatment decisions.[10] A longitudinal study of people with terminal illness found that patients' preferences for involvement changed; initially patients did not want to be involved in the decisions, but as they become more knowledgeable about their condition they wanted to be more involved in the decision making, then as their condition deteriorated they wanted less involvement.[14] This change in preference for involvement was also noted by Hack and colleagues.[15] These studies suggest that there is a need for clinicians to check patient preference during the course of treatment or an illness.

There are also patients who will not want to be involved and prefer the health professional to make the actual decision. Various studies have been undertaken in an attempt to determine which patients want to be involved in clinical decision making and many of the findings are contradictory – for example, some studies suggest that younger people want greater involvement[8,16,17] although this cannot be supported by some other studies.[9,18] What can be surmised is that the wish to participate in clinical decision making is primarily based on individual preferences, which may change over time.

Presentation of information

Information needs to be understood in order for use to be made of it. Regardless of educational level, many people have a limited knowledge about their body – how it works and is constructed. Many people are not aware about the self-limiting nature of common illnesses and a study of patients admitted to a Coronary Care Unit highlighted the public's poor knowledge of health-related issues, with the study identifying that the patients had a comparatively poor awareness of the risk factors of coronary heart disease.[19]

It has also been stated that most people do not have the scientific or statistical understanding 'to make truly informed judgements about complex medical or any other kind of scientific evidence' and the public's reaction, in 1996, to potential risk factors of a range of oral contraceptives is used to illustrate the point.[20] Although there have been criticisms for the way the issue was handled by the government and its medical officers, efforts were made to inform and reassure the public about the risk factors; yet many women panicked and stopped taking the pill and put themselves open to the risks of pregnancy and, in some cases, abortion. These risks were greater than if they had continued taking the pill, but the understanding of relative risk remains at a low level.

Hope highlights that the way in which information is presented makes a difference to what people will actually do.[7] The implication of this for evidence-based care is that a different choice may be made by the patient when the same information is presented in different forms, this is called the 'framing' of information. He provides a simple example of 'this treatment will give you a 5% chance of dying' (the negative frame), compared with 'this treatment gives you a 95% chance of living' (the positive frame) and raises the question of how should information be provided in order to maximise patient choice. The issue of framing with acutely ill cancer patients was studied by O'Connor, who found that if the chance of survival was high, then patients tended to choose that treatment which gave the highest chance of survival whatever the adverse effects.[21] If the chance of survival was low, then patients tended to opt for the treatment with the lowest side effects. Health professionals need to be aware that how they present information to patients can influence their choice and if there is a possibility that how the information is framed would be important, then the same information ought to be presented in different ways in order to help the patient's understanding. But there should not be a deliberate attempt to manipulate the patient's decision through the choice of frame.

Sources of information

There are many sources of health information – relatives and friends, clinicians, support groups, newspapers, magazines, TV and radio, specialist journals, booklets, videos, health help lines, the Internet – but there is little evidence available as to who most needs information. Studies from the monitoring of work by information services, such as telephone help lines, have shown that women, under pensionable age, and people of the higher socio-economic status tend to be the main users of the services. A general public study reflected similar findings in that young or middle aged women of higher social classes were better informed about health issues.[22] The lack of information about health and the health services to black and ethnic minority groups has been highlighted by Hopkins and Bahl,[23] and Buckland stressed that lack of knowledge about where to go to seek information and advice is an issue: 'Individuals may not perceive a need for information if they are unaware that they are lacking such information'.[24] Buckland's study also showed that family, friends and books were the sources most frequently used prior to consultation with a health professional and that information about conditions and illnesses from nursing and medical staff was often limited.[25]

The most common form of information provision is the written word and this is likely to remain so for some time. Various initiatives are in place to produce leaflets/booklets that are evidence based; these include collaborative work between the NHS Centre for Reviews and Dissemination and the Midwives Information and

Resource Services to produce a parallel range of evidence-based leaflets for childbearing women and professionals on general subjects, such as ultrasound scanning, and on topics of more limited interest, such as the management of breech delivery.[26] Another collaboration is between the NHS Centre for Reviews and Dissemination and Bedfordshire Health Authority to adapt, for lay people, the *Effective Health Care* bulletin on glue ear.

Many health organisations have embarked on the production of patient information leaflets and other information packages, such as video and audio tapes. These are frequently used to augment health professionals' verbal information to patients. Although much well-intentioned effort has gone into their development, this is no guarantee that the material will be of good quality and useful. To help overcome the potential variety of quality and usefulness, the Centre for Health Information Quality was established to:

> act as a source of expertise and knowledge for the NHS and patient representative groups on all aspects of patient information with the aim of improving the NHS's competence and capacity to provide good, evidence-based patient information.[27]

The Centre is based at the Help for Health Trust, Winchester and acts as a clearing house and centre of excellence on all aspects of patient information. The development of quality tools to evaluate information for patients, a database of good practice in the creation of good quality patient information and a collection of quality information materials in print and non-print formats are part of its work. In addition, a programme of training for information producers and a network of topic-based patient panels to review available material in the light of needs and priorities of patients are also being undertaken.

The King's Fund, through its Promoting Patient Choice programme, has examined the issues around healthcare partnerships and improving patient choice through information provision and dissemination of information on treatment outcomes by consumer health information services.[28,29]

The Internet has become a source of health information for many members of the general public and health professionals. There are an increasing number of anecdotes from a variety of health professionals about patients who have arrived at a consultation or for treatment with information gleaned from the Internet that they want to discuss, or want to follow. Many professionals have had to say that they were not familiar with the information and wanted time to find the article or conduct a search to assess the evidence. The main concern about the Internet, and not just in the health arena, is that a large proportion of the information available may be incomplete, misleading or plain inaccurate. As discussed in Chapter 4, efforts are being made to assess the quality of health information on the Internet, but many people will be unaware of these and may not have the necessary knowledge to make a judgement about the authenticity of a site. For example, how many members of the general public will be able to determine whether the credentials or affiliations of the authors or contributors are appropriate, let alone whether the research being reported contains all of the required information to determine validity and relevance? There are also concerns that access, or lack of access, to the Internet will disadvantage the vulnerable groups of people who already have limited choice in terms of healthcare.[30]

Critical appraisal skills

Critical appraisal skills workshops are held for members of self-help groups and consumer health information services, which are intended to improve the critical appraisal skills in those who provide information to consumers about healthcare, and to raise awareness about the sources of effectiveness data.[7]

Patient information and the generation of evidence

There are two dimensions to patient involvement in evidence-based healthcare – not only is there a need for the patient to be involved in clinical decision making but it has been argued that consumers need to be involved in determining the issues for research, the focus and design of research and evaluation of evidence.[31] A series of booklets provide an analysis of consumer issues including involvement of consumers in the research agenda, and a report from a workshop on involvement of consumers in local healthcare.[32] There are, potentially, problems of marginalisation of lay people in settings dominated by professionals, and this issue has been addressed by the Cochrane Collaboration in the development of a Consumer

Network.[33] This network is pioneered by the Australian Cochrane Centre with the aim of fostering an environment which will encourage and facilitate consumer input and promote consumer groups' participation in, and use of, systematic reviews.

Evidence-based practice should enhance the quality of information available for patients, enable patients to discriminate between good and poor evidence and start to involve consumers in determining the research agenda so that issues that they believe are important are addressed. Although many patients will want to be involved in the clinical decision-making process, there are still those who, at different stages, may not want to be involved and health professionals will need to remember that the amount of information individual patients want will vary.

References

1 Department of Health (1990) *The Health of the Nation.* HMSO, London.
2 Department of Health (1991) *The Patient's Charter.* HMSO, London.
3 Kempson E (1987) *Informing Health Consumers. a review of consumer health information needs and services.* College of Health British Library, London.
4 Audit Commission (1993) *What Seems to be the Matter? Communication between hospitals and patients.* HMSO, London.
5 Welsh Office (1995) *Towards Evidence Based Practice.* Central Office of Information, Cardiff.
6 NHS Executive (1996) *Promoting Clinical Effectiveness: a framework for action in and through the NHS.* Department of Health, Leeds.
7 Hope T (1996) *Evidence Based Patient Choice.* King's Fund, London.
8 Strull WM, Lo B and Charles G (1984) Do patients want to participate in medical decision making? *Journal of the American Medical Association.* **252**: 2990–4.
9 Johnson JD et al. (1996) Breast cancer patients' personality style, age, and treatment decision making. *Journal of Surgical Oncology.* **63**(3): 183–6.
10 Deber RB (1994) Physicians in healthcare management: 8. The patient–physician partnership: decision making, problem solving and the desire to participate. *Canadian Medical Association Journal.* **151**(4): 423–7.
11 Deber RB, Kraetschmer N and Irvine J (1996) What role do patients

wish to play in treatment decision making? *Archives of Internal Medicine.* **156**(13): 1414–20.

12 Avis M (1994) Choice cuts: an exploratory study of patients' views about the participation in decision making in a day surgery unit. *International Journal of Nursing Studies.* **31**(3): 289–98.

13 Trnobranski PH (1994) Nurse-patient negotiation: assumption or reality? *Journal of Advanced Nursing.* **19**(4): 733–7.

14 Barry B and Henderson A (1996) Nature of decision making in the terminally ill patient. *Cancer Nursing.* **19**(5): 384–91.

15 Hack TF, Degner LF, Farber JM and McWilliams ME (1992) *Communication Between Cancer Patients and Healthcare Professionals: an annotated bibliography.* National Cancer Institute of Canada, Winnipeg.

16 Knobf MT (1994) Decision making for primary breast cancer treatment. *MEDSURG Nursing.* **3**(3): 169–74.

17 Llewellyn-Thomas HA, McGreal MJ and Thiel EC (1995) Cancer patients' decision making and trial-entry preferences: the effects of 'framing' information about short-term toxicity and long-term survival. *Medical Decision Making.* **15**(1): 4–12.

18 Beisecker AE, Helmig L, Graham D and Moore WP (1994) Attitudes of oncologists, oncology nurses and patients from a women's clinic regarding medical decision making for older and younger breast cancer patients. *Gerontologist.* **34**(4): 505–12.

19 Murray PJ (1989) Rehabilitation information and health beliefs in the post-coronary patient: do we meet their information needs? *Journal of Advanced Nursing.* **14**: 686–93.

20 Grayson L (1997) *Evidence Based Medicine: an overview and guide to the literature.* British Library, London.

21 O'Connor A (1989) Effects of framing and level of probability on patients' preferences for cancer chemotherapy. *Journal of Clinical Epidemiology.* **42**: 119–26.

22 Chamy M, Klein R, Lewis PA and Tipping GK (1990) Britain's new market model of general practice: do consumers know enough to make it work? *Health Policy.* **14**: 243–52.

23 Hopkins A and Bahl V (1993) *Access to Healthcare for People from Black and Ethnic Minorities.* Royal College of Physicians, London.

24 Buckland S (1994) Unmet needs for health information: a literature review. *Health Libraries Review.* **11**: 82–95.

25 Buckland A (1995) *Unmet Needs for Health Information: Report to Nuffield Provincial Hospitals.* Help for Health Trust, Winchester.

26 Oliver S, Rajan L, Turner H *et al.* (1996) Informed choice for users of health services: views on ultrasonography leaflets of women in early pregnancy, midwives and ultrasonographers. *British Medical Journal.* **313**: 1251–3.

27 Department of Health (1996) *Primary Care: delivering the future.* Cmnd 3512. HMSO, London.

28 Farrell C and Gilbert H (1996) *Healthcare Partnerships: debates and strategies for increasing patient involvement in healthcare and health services.* King's Fund, London.

29 Buckland S and Gann B (1994) *Dissemination of Information on Treatment Outcomes by Consumer Health Information Services: Report to King's Fund.* Help for Health Trust, Winchester.

30 Dick R, Steen EB and Detmer DE (eds) (1997) *The Computer-based Patient Record: an essential technology for health care* (Revised edition). National Academy Press, Washington DC.

31 Oliver S (1995) How can health service users contribute to the NHS research and development programme? *British Medical Journal.* 310: 1318–20.

32 NHS Executive (1995) *Consumers and Research in the NHS: consumer issues within the NHS.* NHS Executive/R&D Directorate, Leeds.

33 Bastian H (1994) *The Power of Sharing Knowledge: consumer participation in the Cochrane Collaboration.* Cochrane Collaboration Paper. Available via *http://hiru.mcmaster.ca/cochrane/default.htm*

8 Clinical audit

Clinical audit is an integral part of evidence-based practice – it provides the mechanism for checking that practice is achieving the desired results; it can highlight areas for further research; and findings from well-conducted audit can improve knowledge and replace opinion with evidence. Clinical audit can also highlight failure to apply the results of research; deficiencies in skills and knowledge in clinical care; and may reveal quality assurance deficiencies, such as incompleteness of clinical records and limitations of clinical coding.

What is audit?

Audit is a process 'used by health professionals to assess, evaluate and improve the care of patients in a systematic way, to enhance their health and quality of life'.[1] It can be undertaken by the individual health professional in order to review their own work; a team of health professionals, such as a practice or a ward team, can undertake an audit of their own care; there can be an audit by peers, or by others external to the health professionals concerned. The essential features of audit have been identified by several authors and can be summarised as:[2,3]

- identifying the problem or topic for audit
- defining standards, criteria, targets or protocols for good practice against which performance can be compared
- systematic gathering of objective evidence about performance
- comparing results against standards
- identifying deficiencies and possible solutions
- implementing planned change
- monitoring the effects of the planned change.

Although audits have been undertaken within the health service for many years, the Griffiths Inquiry (1983) did note that evaluation of clinical practices was not common.[4] In 1985, the Royal College of General Practitioners asked doctors to define objectives for patient care, to assess their performance against the objectives and, where appropriate, to make changes to practice.[5] However, the main emphasis on audit activities within the NHS followed the 1989 paper, *Medical Audit: Working Paper No. 6, Working for Patients.*[6] Initially, audit activities were targeted and funded at individual professional groups, then multiprofessional issues were the focus for clinical audit. The original White Paper definition of medical audit has been amended to reflect the evolution of thinking to:

> the systematic critical analysis of the quality of care, involving the procedures and processes used for diagnosis, intervention and treatment, the use of resources and the resulting outcome and quality of life as assessed by both professionals and patients.[7]

Audit should thus have a powerful role in evidence-based care if undertaken effectively, as it generates objective evidence as to what is happening locally in care delivery matched against what should be happening. This should, therefore, be powerful evidence for the review and improvement of care, but there must be a commitment to act upon it. However, to achieve this relevance audit is demanding in the way it harnesses health information, as it requires both national and local information and their matching together according to audit information principles. The national information is drawn from best practice evidence, as described in earlier chapters of this book, but this needs to be turned wherever possible into numeric measures in the form of standards or targets. It is important to differentiate whether such standards are absolute or normative if the audit results are to contain correct interpretation of practice quality.[8] The data on local care activity and results are obtained from operational sources as indicated in the following section. The two are then matched together, and this process of comparison requires that common data definitions and formats are used, which itself can be difficult but essential.

This systematic review of the quality of care provided can take place after the episode of care has been completed (retrospective audit), or undertaken while the patient is still receiving care (concurrent audit). When planning audit, decisions are required about how frequently data needs to be collected and what methods and tools should be used to ensure that good quality data is available. Data collection and verification can be costly, thus there may need to be a balance between using routinely available data and specially collected data. To achieve as high a quality of data as is feasible for audit, data needs to be collected as near source as possible, by appropriate staff who understand and value the data, and collected at the appropriate level for the audit being carried out.[9] Improvement to the quality of data within the NHS, especially that recorded in patients' healthcare records, has been the focus of several Audit Commission reports,[10,11] and many trusts have taken action to review what data is actually collected and improve the quality of patient records and other routinely collected data. Audit, however, needs to be informed by all relevant data not just data from the patient record, and this may necessitate the collection of data from other routine sources, such as details from records held in operating theatres about staff in attendance during specific operations, and may, occasionally, require specially collected data. What is important is that the method used to audit a particular aspect of care should be capable of measuring what it is intended to measure.

Audit in practice

Health organisations have invested a lot of time, money and energies into undertaking audit, but many health professionals still display a lack of enthusiasm towards formal audit. Some health professionals are likely to say that as analyses of the benefits of audit programmes have found it difficult to identify benefits to patients, then they have sufficient work to do without including an activity that has little relevance to patient care.[12,13] Earnshaw argues that audit should not, necessarily, be held to blame for the disappointing findings, but that 'Audit is only a tool and its failure to achieve measurable benefit is a reflection on the way it has been undertaken, rather than the concept itself'.[14]

A survey to evaluate the development of audit has shown that there was a wide variation in the way in which audit programmes had been implemented and that there had only been a slow move towards multiprofessional audit.[15] The Clinical Standards Advisory Group (CSAG) study into clinical effectiveness also noted that there were shortfalls in the way several audits had been undertaken.[16]

How can an organisation, or a clinical team, determine how well their audits were carried out, or identify what criteria are required for an audit to be of high quality? The National Centre for Clinical Audit has produced a Clinical Audit Action Pack. The framework covers aspects such as how and why the topic was chosen, how well based the audit standards are in the research evidence, whether the objectives were measurable, how rigorously the data was collected, the evaluation of actual and ideal practice and the use made of the information to plan and implement improvements and whether actions were taken and re-audited. Time is needed to complete the full audit cycle, with Auplish suggesting that an average audit cycle takes between 12 to 18 months, i.e. to set up the programme, collect, analyse and present data, make recommendations for changes, and then to re-audit after sufficient time has been allowed to implement the changes.[17] Many audit programmes have started off the cycle, but not always provided the opportunity to re-audit to ensure that any planned changes have been implemented and are achieving the expected results.

In his article, Earnshaw comments that it is often difficult interesting junior doctors in undertaking or presenting audit projects.[14] Walshe and Buttery had noted that research activities were perceived by trainees to have advantages in terms of publications and presentations, whereas audit projects were perceived as having little value.[18] The CSAG study noted that many doctors saw audit as 'an empty exercise imposed on them as an NHS fad'.[16] However, the other clinical professions were less cynical but were frustrated over the lack of genuinely multidisciplinary audit. The other clinical professions felt that audit tended to be a medically dominated activity which focused on data gathering rather than on making changes. As highlighted earlier in this chapter, clinical audit is an integral part of evidence-based care as it provides the mechanism for checking that practice is achieving the desired results. The findings from well-conducted audit can also improve knowledge and help with replacing opinion with evidence, as well as identifying areas for further research. Health professionals, therefore, ought to have a positive attitude towards clinical audit.

Promoting a positive change in professional attitudes towards clinical audit is one of the main objectives of the National Centre for Clinical Audit.[19] The centre was established in 1995 and is a partnership of 14 professional organisations. The partnership is led by the British Medical Association and the Royal College of Nursing, and includes organisations such as the British Dietetics Association, British Orthoptic Association, British Psychological Society, Chartered Society of Physiotherapy, National Institute for Social Work, Royal College of Speech and Language Therapists, Society and College of Radiographers, and Society of Chiropodists and

Podiatrists. It is intended that the Centre will serve as a model for a collaborative approach between health professional groups. The partners' existing networks, both with individuals and organisations, should make dissemination of information about the Centre easier and the networks should provide access to current clinical audit activities.

The first task of the Centre was the development of the criteria for clinical audit and production of the Clinical Audit Action Pack. It is anticipated that by having criteria there will be less diversity of approach towards clinical audit and that it will provide a framework between the professions. The criteria for clinical audit have also been incorporated into the record design for the database of examples of good audit practice. Publications on clinical audit and quality in healthcare, information about meetings, courses and contacts will also be maintained. The Centre currently provides a help desk during office hours. In 1999, the National Centre for Clinical Audit became part of the new National Institute for Clinical Excellence (*see* Chapter 9).

Even though the National Centre for Clinical Audit exists to improve implementation of clinical audit, there is also a two year project, *Action on Clinical Audit*, that is 'devised to unravel the complex relationships that seem to render audit unworkable'.[20] Teams from 22 trusts are working together and conducting a systematic analyses of the stages of audit and identifying barriers.

User involvement in clinical audit

It has been recommended that patients should be more fully involved in audit[7,21] and there has been some progress towards this with patient representatives from the Consumers Association becoming members of trust clinical audit committees and primary care medical audit advisory groups, and a few places have actual involvement of patients on the audit team.[22]

Many patients are probably unaware that audits are undertaken, and health professionals need to consider the best ways of involving patients in identifying which topics should be audited, setting the standards, designing the audit and drawing up recommendations after analysis of the obtained data, as well as in the dissemination of findings.

Outcomes

The early work on quality of healthcare focused on the structure and process elements of Donabedian's structure, process and outcome framework,[23] even though outcome is considered 'the most relevant indicator of the quality of patient care and an essential balance to performance indicators relating entirely to process and cost'.[24] Morbidity and mortality statistics, complications and patient satisfaction were the most common outcome measures, but more recently work has taken place to improve methods for measuring outcomes and a national clearing house for assessing health service outcomes has been established.[25] However, defining and measuring outcomes can be difficult, costly and time consuming. Gulliford and Orchard comment that the coding and recording of routine patient data within most NHS trusts is likely to prove inadequate for use in outcome measures.[26,27] Paper records are not well organised, or sufficiently structured, which makes them difficult to use for information retrieval and analysis. Occasionally, process measures are employed as proxies for health outcomes when the latter are unavailable.[28] For example, if clinical trials or meta-analyses have determined that a certain treatment, such as giving heart attack patients streptokinase within 24 hours, correlates closely to patient outcome, then it is valid to measure the speed of administration of this treatment as a proxy for the outcome. It is anticipated that the introduction of electronic patient records will enable data to be more easily retrieved and analysed. Lock, however, states that '. . . the range of outcomes that might arise from computer systems is potentially huge, and yet no measure of outcome has been universally recognised'.[29]

Role of audit in evidence-based care

Well-conducted clinical audit has a vital role to play in evidence-based care. A clinical team may have started off their quest for information about best practice either from the findings of an audit or from their own concerns about whether the care being given for a specific clinical problem is actually the best. Following the search and appraisal of the information, the team may have identified changes that they want to implement. The plan for change needs to include the undertaking of an audit to check not only that the planned changes are being implemented, but also whether the expected results from the interventions are being achieved. The evidence obtained during the search will be used to set the standards for the audit.

Obtaining the relevant data to determine whether the standards set are being achieved can be a major difficulty when undertaking audit. Incompleteness of the clinical record is a common problem as health professionals have omitted to record all information, or information is recorded but it is illegible.[10,11] As part of the change implementation plan, the clinical team may decide that staff have to pay specific attention to their record keeping and ensure that it is up to the required standard. As already discussed in this chapter, few outcome measurement tools are available and process measures may have to be used. There are still only a few trusts that have electronic patient records, and most trusts will need to overcome the practical difficulties of identifying the relevant records and then finding not just the actual record, but also the relevant data from the records. This activity can be very time consuming.

The search for best practice may only have identified Level IV or III evidence (as discussed in Chapter 3). The clinical team may have decided to implement this but to monitor, within a specific time, whether the expected results are being achieved. If the audit findings are positive, then the team is likely to be more confident that the most appropriate care is being delivered. Even if the evidence was Level I or II, the team may have been concerned that the study patient group may not have been exactly the same as those they care for and want to check that the interventions do achieve the expected results.

In the future, NHS trusts will be expected to have clinical audit systems in place in all clinical departments to ensure that good practice, ideas and innovations can be introduced and evaluated. Trusts will be expected to undertake local audits and participate in the current four National Confidential Enquiries and other external audit programmes. Clinical audit activities will need to become part of the processes for assuring the quality of clinical care in the endeavour to deliver the same level of service for the same level of need to all patients.[30]

References

1   Irvine D and Irvine S (eds) (1997) *Making Sense of Audit* (2nd ed). Radcliffe Medical Press, Oxford.

2   Hughes J and Humphrey C (1990) *Medical Audit in General Practice: a practical guide to the literature.* King Edward's Hospital Fund for London, London.

3   Malby B (1995) *Clinical Audit for Nurses and Therapists.* Scutari Press, London.

4   Department of Health and Social Security (1983) *NHS Management Inquiry: Griffiths NHS Management Inquiry Report.* Department of Health and Social Security, London.

5   Royal College of General Practitioners (1985) *Quality in General Practice.* Policy statement 2. RCGP, London.

6   Department of Health (1989) *Medical Audit: Working Paper No. 6, Working for Patients.* HMSO, London.

7   Welsh Office (1996) *Framework for the Development of Multi-Professional Clinical Audit in Wales.* Welsh Office, Cardiff.

8   Rigby M (1998) Consumer Orientation and Service Quality. In: M Rigby, EM Ross and NT Begg (eds) *Management for Child Health Services.* Chapman and Hall, London.

9   NHS Executive, Greenhalgh & Company Ltd (1996) *Using Clinical Information in Integrated Healthcare.* H Charlesworth, Huddersfield.

10 Audit Commission (1995) *Setting the Records Straight: a study of hospital medical records.* HMSO, London.

11 Audit Commission (1997) *Comparing Notes: a study of information management in community trusts.* Audit Commission Publications, London.

12 Eagle CJ, Davies JM and Pagenkopt D (1994) The cost of an established quality assurance programme: is it worth it? *Canadian Journal of Anaesthesia.* **41**: 813–17.

13 Johnson DS and Faux JC (1997) The hidden cost of audit. *Annals of the Royal College of Surgeons England.* **79**: 12–14 (Suppl).

14 Earnshaw JJ (1997) Auditing audit: the cost of the emperor's new clothes. *British Journal of Hospital Medicine.* **58**(5): 198–2.

15 Buttery Y, Walshe K, Coles J and Bennett J (1994) *The Development of Audit: findings of a national survey of healthcare provider units in England.* CASPE Research, London.

16 Clinical Standards Advisory Group (1998) *Clinical Effectiveness: Report on clinical effectiveness using stroke care as an example.* The Stationery Office, London.

17 Auplish S (1997) Using clinical audit to promote evidence-based

medicine and clinical effectiveness: an overview of experience. *Journal of Evaluation in Clinical Practice.* **3**(1): 77–82.

18 Walshe K and Buttery Y (1995) Measuring the impact of audit and quality improvement programmes. *Journal of the Association of Quality in Healthcare.* **2**: 138–47.

19 Smith JE (1996) The National Centre for Clinical Audit: the first stage. *Journal of Clinical Effectiveness.* **1**(1): 3–4.

20 Berger A (1998) Why doesn't audit work? *British Medical Journal.* **316**: 875–6.

21 NHS Executive (1996) *Clinical Audit in the NHS.* Department of Health, Leeds.

22 Kelson M and Redpath L (1996) Promoting user involvement in clinical audit: surveys of audit committees in primary and secondary care. *Journal of Clinical Effectiveness.* **1**(1): 14–18.

23 Donabedian A (1966) Evaluating the quality of medical care. *Milbank Memorial Fund Quarterly.* **44**(2): 166–206.

24 Royal College of Physicians (1989) *Medical Audit: A First Report: What, why and how?* Royal College of Physicians, London.

25 Long AF, Dixon P, Hall R *et al.* (1993) The outcome agenda: contribution of the UK clearing house on health outcomes. *Quality in Health Care.* **2**(1): 49–52.

26 Gulliford MC (1992) Evaluating prognostic factors: implications for measurement of healthcare outcomes. *Journal of Epidemiology and Community Health.* **46**(4): 323–6.

27 Orchard C (1994) Comparing healthcare outcomes. *British Medical Journal.* **308**: 1493–6.

28 Mant J and Hicks N (1995) Detecting differences in quality of care: the sensitivity of measures of process and outcome in treating acute myocardial infarction. *British Medical Journal.* **311**: 793–6.

29 Lock C (1996) What value do computers provide to NHS hospitals? *British Medical Journal.* **312**: 1407–10.

30 Secretary of State for Health (1997) *A First Class Service: quality in the new NHS.* Cmnd Paper 3807. Department of Health, London.

9   And what next?

There has been much activity towards implementing evidence-based care. Many trusts and health authorities have been involved with projects, usually focused on a single clinical topic or area with many of the topics being selected from those featured in the *Effective Health Care* bulletins (discussed in Chapter 4).[1] The bulletins have undertaken the searching for and appraisal of the evidence, so that the project teams have been able to consider these in light of their local circumstances. They have then planned how to ensure that the effective care is implemented, and monitored as to whether the expected results have been realised. Frequently, the projects have been undertaken by health professionals who are enthusiasts of evidence-based care and who have put in some personal time and a lot of commitment to ensure the projects are successful.

Although projects are a useful starting point, there is also a need for trusts and health authorities to have a strategy for moving forward beyond small projects. The King's Fund PACE programme suggests that for improvements resulting from these small 'demonstration' projects to be sustained and replicated, there needs to be a wider process of organisational change.[2] Waters argues that there is fragmentation of activities such as guideline, protocols and care pathways production, research and development efforts, and clinical audit which are 'commonly unfocused and unrelated to the practical demands of everyday clinical practice'[3] – trusts need to co-ordinate these under the umbrella of a clinical effectiveness department or directorate.

Structured approach to quality

The latest White Papers emphasised that all patients in the NHS should receive the same level of service and quality of care for the same level of need.[4,5] NHS organisations will be expected to adopt a structured approach to quality and will be accountable for improving the quality of their services. This new framework has been termed 'clinical governance'. Clear lines of responsibility and accountability, clear policies and a comprehensive programme of quality improvement activity, such as clinical audit and evidence-based practice, have been identified as key components of the framework. The chief executive will have ultimate responsibility for assuring the quality of services and a designated senior clinician will be responsible for ensuring that systems for clinical governance are in place and monitoring their effectiveness. The systems for clinical governance in each trust or healthcare organisation will emerge with time and experience, since detailed blueprints were not provided by government when introducing policy, but the opportunity exists to ensure co-ordination of the various activities relating to evidence-based care. However, it needs to be remembered that:

> As well as building on organisational influences of clinical quality, true clinical governance will not be achieved without the willing commitment of individual practitioners to high standards of practice.[6]

For the first time national standards will be drawn up through joint working between the professionals and the health departments, and set through National Service Frameworks and the National Institute for Clinical Excellence (NICE).[4,5] The frameworks are intended to specify how services can best be organised for patients with specific conditions and the standards that services will have to meet. The first framework developed in Wales is for cervical screening which became available in the autumn of 1998 for health authorities to plan for implementation through their health improvement programmes.[5]

The CSAG stroke care study identified that the evidence available for guiding clinical practice was 'less robust than we had expected'.[7] Other recent articles have also expressed concerns about the availability of information on treatment of individual patients.[8–11] It is proposed that NICE will help to clarify, both for patients and professionals, which treatments work best and those which do not. The Institute will be responsible for the appraisal and production of guidance and its dissemination to the NHS. It is also expected that in the course of its work the Institute will identify gaps in evidence and these will be addressed through the UK NHS Research and Development programmes. The National Confidential Enquiry into Perioperative Deaths (NCEPOD), Confidential Enquiry into Stillbirths and Deaths in Infancy (CESDI), Confidential Enquiry into Maternal Deaths (CEMD) and Confidential Inquiry into Suicide and Homicide by People with Mental Illness (CISH) will be brought together under the umbrella of NICE and results from their findings will feed into appropriate guidance and standard setting. NICE is intended to provide a single focus for the appraisal of evidence and production of clinical guidance, and for the first time the government, working with the professional organisations, will systematically appraise medical technologies before they are introduced into the NHS.

As a Special Health Authority, NICE's membership incorporates the health professions, the NHS, academics, health economists and patient representatives. It brings together a range of functions previously undertaken by a number of different groups – the National Centre for Clinical Audit, the National Prescribing Centre appraisals and bulletins, the Department of Health funded National Guidelines Programme and Professional Audit Programme, Effectiveness Bulletins and the clinical guidance contained in PRODIGY (a computer aided decision support system for GPs to assist in their prescribing practice). The activities of NICE are funded from the resources allocated for the previous activities.

The quality agenda is seen as a 10 year plan and the emphasis on quality of healthcare has been welcomed; however, concerns have been expressed about the lack of new funds and the risk that the drive for quality will not be high on everyone's agenda because of the demands of other ongoing changes such as setting up primary care groups and restructuring acute services.[12]

Continuing education

Placing clinical practice on a more scientific basis is dependent upon successfully accessing reliable evidence.[13] The role of electronic databases was discussed in Chapter 4; however, many health professionals have limited experience of using these databases.[14,15] The skills of undertaking a literature search are being incorporated into many junior doctor orientation programmes as well as becoming part of short courses on research methods. However, these skills need to be used after the initial training for the health professional to become proficient.

Some organisations are now making information resources, such as MedLine and Cochrane Library databases, more available to clinicians at, or close to, their workplace through computer networks.[1] Clinical guidelines used by the organisation, hospital formulary and junior doctor handbooks are also being placed on the hospital intranet. Many of these organisations are also undertaking studies into the effectiveness of using this approach.

Managers need to understand that health professionals practising evidence-based care require time to undertake the literature searches, appraise the evidence, plan and monitor the required change. Doctors have 'protected' time for continuing education, but it is rare for nurses and the professions allied to medicine to have any protected time. If multiprofessional, evidence-based care is to be widely implemented then the strategies must consider how this can be done without health professionals having to devote a lot of their own time to the various activities.

Workshops and courses have been provided to improve the skills of undertaking a literature search and appraising the evidence. However, these are just a few of the skills required by practitioners to ensure that effective healthcare interventions are adopted in practice, and ineffective or harmful interventions are abandoned. Health professionals also need to understand how to manage, and adapt to, change.[16] Change is the process of bringing about an alteration or substituting one way of behaving for another. Much has been written on change and the one thing all writers agree on is that change is not easy and there are various stages that all people undergo which must be recognised and supported for the change to be successful.[17,18,19] Change should be planned and systematically implemented and if change, such as implementing evidence-based care, is going to be implemented in a multidisciplinary team, then all members of the team need to be involved and viewed as equals in achieving that change.[20]

Evidence based care has highlighted the need for health professionals to keep up-to-date and adopt 'a process of lifelong, self-directed learning'.[21] Lifelong learning has also been identified as a requirement for many other jobs. It has been argued that there are now few jobs that can be carried out solely on the knowledge acquired at school and university, and Handy comments that individuals need to assess and acknowledge their own deficiencies and update their personal portfolio of skills and experience in response to new technology and the changing requirements of the job.[22]

The government has emphasised that UK citizens need to become lifelong learners, and the White Papers identify the need for an organisational culture that values lifelong learning.[4,5] Continuing professional development (CPD) is seen as the process of lifelong learning for all individuals and teams which will enable professionals to fulfil their potential while 'meeting the needs of patients and delivering the health outcomes and healthcare priorities of the NHS'.[5] Many health professionals already agree their individual development plan during their annual performance review process; however, by April 2000 all health professionals will be required to have a personal development plan (PDP) which identifies the professional and service needs. It should be remembered that learning opportunities arise not only on courses but also 'on-the-job' and that the roles of mentoring and supervision are likely to expand.

Optimal care: a personal and corporate responsibility

Individual health professionals, clinical teams, professional bodies, and healthcare managers all have an important part to play in ensuring that the care delivered to patients is based on the best possible evidence. The range of skills required is wide, skills not just relating to information seeking, retrieval, appraisal and dissemination, but also to planning and monitoring the care. Interpersonal skills to ensure true multiprofessional team working and the appropriate participation of patients in their care are also needed. The organisation should provide an environment that supports and facilitates evidence-based care. As the CSAG study highlighted, although there are shortfalls of evidence available for determining what is the best care, there are also many instances where health professionals were not aware of the available evidence. The implementation of these interventions would increase the proportion of clinical services shown by evidence to be effective and help to reduce the inequality of provision of care to patients throughout the NHS.

Education of all health professionals focuses on the importance of making clinical decisions based on sound evidence, though only recently has the need for lifelong learning to update with new knowledge been adequately recognised. Hippocrates emphasised practice being based on doing good and not causing harm (a challenging double test of applied knowledge). Ethical duties require appropriate treatment for each patient, whilst legal responsibility hinges on 'reasonableness' of care – both concepts inextricably linked to use of practice proven to be safe and effective, of which the clinician therefore has duty to be aware.

The NHS was established to deliver healthcare in a rational, efficient and fair way across the UK. With the expanding initiatives to identify and promote best practice, the opportunity exists for individual health professionals, clinical teams, professional bodies and healthcare managers to work together and co-ordinate the various activities to promote adoption of evidence-based care. No one person or small group of people will achieve a reduction in the inequalities of care for all UK citizens, but no team can optimise its care unless all members espouse this goal, and commit themselves personally. The process of posing clinical questions, systematically locating, appraising and using the best evidence in conjunction with clinical judgement and experience, and monitoring the effectiveness of care by clinical teams will make a difference to the quality of care delivered to the patients in each locality by every clinician. If all clinical teams took this approach, then the inequalities of care would diminish. Only by understanding and harnessing the information increasingly being made available will this fundamental objective be achieved.

References

1   Walshe K and Ham C (1997) Who's acting on the evidence? *Health Service Journal.* **107**: 22–5.
2   Dunning M (1996) *From Project to Mainstream.* PACE Discussion Paper. King's Fund, London.
3   Waters E (1997) Improving clinical effectiveness. *Journal of Evaluation in Clinical Practice.* **3**(4): 255–64.
4   Secretary of State for Health (1997) *A First Class Service: quality in the new NHS.* Cmnd Paper 3807. Department of Health, London.
5   Welsh Office (1998) *Quality Care and Clinical Excellence.* Welsh Office, Cardiff.
6   Chambers R (1998) *Clinical Effectiveness Made Easy: first thoughts on clinical governance.* Radcliffe Medical Press, Oxford.
7   Clinical Standards Advisory Group (1998) *Clinical Effectiveness: Report on clinical effectiveness using stroke care as an example.* The Stationery Office, London.
8   Lau J, Ioannidis JPA and Schmid CH (1998) Summing up evidence: one answer is not always enough. *The Lancet.* **351**: 123–7.

9   Haynes B and Haines A (1998) Getting research findings into practice: barriers and bridges to evidence-based clinical practice. *British Medical Journal.* **317**: 273–6.

10 Sheldon TA, Guyatt GH and Haines A (1998) Getting research into practice: when to act on the evidence. *British Medical Journal.* **317**: 139–42.

11 Godlee F (1998) Getting evidence into practice needs the right resources and the right organisation. *British Medical Journal.* **317**: 6.

12 Healy P (1998) NICE work if you can fund it. *Health Service Journal.* **108**: 12–13.

13 Freemantle N and Watt I (1994) Dissemination: implementing the findings of research. *Health Libraries Review.* **11**: 133–7.

14 Meah S, Luker KA and Cullum NA (1996) An exploration of midwives' attitudes to research and perceived barriers to research utilisation. *Midwifery.* **12**: 73–84.

15 Olatunbosun OA, Edouard L and Pierson RA (1998) Physicians' attitudes towards evidence based obstetric practice: a questionnaire survey. *British Medical Journal.* **316**: 365–6.

16 Haines AP (1996) The science of perpetual change. *British Journal of General Practice.* **46**: 115–19.

17 Bennis W, Benne K and Chin R (1976) *The Planning of Change* (3rd ed). Holt, Reinhart & Winston Inc., London.

18 Broome A (1990) *Managing Change.* Macmillan, London.

19 Lewin K (1951) *Field Theory in Social Science.* Tavistock, London.

20 Malby B (1995) *Clinical Audit for Nurses and Therapists.* Scutari Press, London.

21 Sackett DL, Richardson WS, Rosenberg W and Haynes RB (1997) *Evidence-based Medicine: how to practice and teach EBM.* Churchill Livingstone, Edinburgh.

22 Handy C (1995) *Beyond Certainty: the changing worlds of organisations.* Hutchinson, London.

Index